TALK
DOES NOT COOK THE RICE

TALK
DOES NOT COOK THE RICE

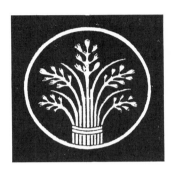

A COMMENTARY ON THE TEACHING
OF AGNI YOGA

by Guru R.H.H.
compiled and edited by his disciple

Samuel Weiser, Inc.
York Beach, Maine

First published in 1982 by   9/84

Samuel Weiser, Inc.
P.O. Box 612
York Beach, Maine 03910

ISBN 0-87728-530-6

Library of Congress Catalog Card No.: 81-70390

Printed in the U.S.A.

Contents

(An alphabetical subject index begins on page 197).

Foreword

The New Age of Light and Illumination which began in September 1936 also saw the rebirth of an ancient yet "new as tomorrow" philosophy, called Agni Yoga. This philosophy is not a religion but a "Teaching of Living Ethics"—the Teaching of the Lord Maitreya.

To quote Helena Roerich, Mother of Agni Yoga, "It is a philosophy given to humanity by the Great Teachers of the White Brotherhood who simply wish to help those who have a desire to broaden their consciousness and to give answers to many of life's problems; answers which religion through thousands of years of existence has failed to give. The books of this Teaching of Life, in their cosmic span of thought, actually give answers to all questions."

The first teacher to be sent out by the Brotherhood, to bring this Teaching to humanity, was Nicholas Roerich. His disciple, our Beloved Guru, RHH, began his mission in San Francisco and later moved on to Los Angeles and New York and finally to an Ashram in upstate New York. As the students and disciples came to this Teaching, and the work spread throughout the United States, Canada and Europe, it became impossible for Guru to be in all these places simultaneously and so his classes were recorded on tape.

This book is a transcription of tapes from over two hundred classes held between 1967 and 1971. Its purpose is to make Guru's commentary on The Teaching available to everyone in a readily accessible form.

He often made the statement, "You don't know your subject until you can explain it simply." As you consult this book for the answers to your questions or just for knowledge and enlightenment, it is immediately apparent that he knew his material. The most abstract and complex esoteric concepts are clearly explained, through illustration and example, so that all who read his words can know and understand.

In editing these tapes every effort has been made to minimize repetition; however, some repetition is necessary as it relates to the over seven hundred eighty subjects discussed.

Guru's unique individuality and style of expression has been maintained throughout. He taught, not as from a lecture platform, but in the intimacy of private homes with his students and disciples seated around him, ofttimes at his feet. He is no longer with us in the physical body, having departed this incarnation on November 4, 1976, but those of us who were privileged to sit in his presence and listen to his words of wisdom, heard with the heart and not the ear, and to read these words in like manner will put you in touch once again with his fiery essence.

Many, many times Guru would say, "The only thing of real value in this life is wisdom," and "Wisdom is the only thing you can take with you from lifetime to lifetime." Within these pages you will find that wisdom which is "your birthright and your heritage," a gift given to you out of love, from Guru RHH.

God Bless...
By his disciple

AGNI YOGA

1. Agni Yoga is the Yoga of Fire, the creative fire of enthusiasm. It is a combination of Bhakti Yoga, the yoga of impersonal love that Christ came to teach; Karma Yoga, which is service; and Raja Yoga, or the yoga of mind—the idea being that knowledge is of no value unless it is put to work. Together with these three forms of yoga, Agni is based on Theosophy and the Mahatmas and their tireless energies to help humanity. The basic idea is that when one becomes enlightened one attains wisdom, but this is not the wisdom we learn out of books. You find wisdom and the way to use it within yourself through the God Channel, which ties in with all religions.

We believe all religions are one. We are born on this planet in many countries and speak many languages, but we are one world and we are one people. There is no such thing as a higher and lower birth. All people are born with a spirit–consciousness and if we can work as a Brotherhood, then we can function as a citizen of the world. Religion is like an apple pie. Each religion is represented as a sliver of that pie. Be greedy for God and want the whole pie. As the Hindus put it, God is the sea and we are each a dewdrop. How can you separate the dewdrop from the sea? You can't. All is one. All the races, all the different denominations are one, because Truth is one. You look around the room and there are many lights giving illumination, yet the light that shines from each individual lamp is the same light that shines from all the lamps together. We bow to God in every form and every religion, because the same Truth is found in all religions. For instance, they all have the Ten Commandments. Actually your Cosmic Laws are the Ten Commandments. They have been given by Moses, by Christ, by Mohammed and by Buddha. They are the same Ten Commandments, only worded in a different way. Moses said, "Thou shalt not kill." Buddha said, "Kill not the meanest thing upon its upward way."

The Upanishads and Vedas are about eight to ten thousand years old and Agni is mentioned in both. Agni is one of the most ancient yogas, yet it is as modern as tomorrow. It's complicated and the most difficult form of yoga that exists. Yoga means "union with God," and this is one path to the realization of God Consciousness.

Agni Yoga or any esoteric order will always meet in homes in small groups so that no political organization can gain control of it nor any group control it or use it for power. There is no money and no bookkeeping. The number one rule in any esoteric or occult Teaching is that there is no fee, no initiation fee or anything like that. The moment there is money involved and you try to sell it like meat and potatoes in the market place it is no longer esoteric. It can't be, because the Teaching is given out of love and received out of love and that's the only way it can be exchanged.

When the Teaching refers to the new ones, this means new people coming into the Teaching for the first time.

You see, this is another wonderful thing. The Hierarchy says, "We send you the people." Whoever comes is sent because no one is ever invited. They say, "Set up your shop, your magnet, by the side of the road and we send you the people. Some will come and look in the window, some will come in the door and tarry awhile, and others will come and remain forever, but it matters not, for if not in this life, then in the next or the next or the next." The important thing is that whoever comes, it is not by accident. Never! This again as Christ said, "Once you have touched the hem of the robe you are never the same." This is true; the hem of the robe being any form of Teaching.

In New York we have very large classes. Always someone will come out and say, you must organize. They go around and make a list of all the names and addresses and phone numbers and they give it to me and I throw it in the wastebasket. This is no good. This is organization and you are doing it. The other way, the Hierarchy is doing it, and you are just sitting there cooperating with them. It is an organization—yes—but on the inner plane. On the outer plane it is completely disorganized, but on the inner plane it is highly organized. The organization is in the hearts of men and that's why the Teaching is always given in the homes. It will never be given in public.

The Agni Yoga classes are held every Tuesday and Thursday at 8:30 P.M., and wherever you are you attend. We have groups in Trenton, New Jersey; in Mt. Vernon, New York; in Staten Island; in New York City; in Atlantic City; in Philadelphia; in Denver; in Taos, New Mexico; in San Antonio, Texas; in Los Angeles; in San Jose, California; in El Sobrante, California; in San Francisco; in Toronto, Canada; Golden, British Columbia; Vancouver, British Columbia; in Oregon; Rome; Paris; Brussels; London—these groups meet on Tuesday and Thursday night and this is why we are making these recordings on tape. The tapes go all over to the various groups and people can play them and work with the Teaching in this way. Tuesday and Thursday night and this is why we are making these occult Teachings work with their Mahatmas. All esoteric orders work closely with their Mahatma.

2. Every hundred years the Mahatmas try to bring the Teaching of wisdom to people in a form they will accept.

First they tried Spiritualism, but when They saw the nonsense that was going on and the interference of the lower astral, plus the fact the mediums couldn't control it, They knew this didn't work. Many people became frightened because there were unethical people who were involved emotionally with spirits who had passed over, so They withdrew.

Then They tried Theosophy. They offered all kinds of proof to people that so-called miracles were an everyday occurrence.

There is an interesting story of an instance that occurred at the time the Mahatmas were trying to get the Theosophical Society started in England. There was a very large dinner party at which the Master M. told Madame Blavatsky to sit at the table and allow each person to ask any question or any favor they wanted and the Mahatmas would grant them their wish. The second lady, when asked, said, "Yes, I lost a broach of emeralds and diamonds on the Riviera twenty-six years ago and I would like it back." M. said, "This will take a little while so go on to the next person," and while they received their request the answer came: "Go out into the rose garden (it was the middle of winter); call the gardener and ask him to dig up a certain rose tree in the center of the garden. Tell him to dig down under the frozen roots and there you will find the pin." They did this and returned her broach wrapped in paper. She said, "This is a fraud. It cannot be." But, she had the pin back.

At this same time the Mahatmas levitated the scientist Hume up six stories outside a building and in through the window and he said, "It's mass hypnosis." These are two examples of what They went through to prove that these things do exist, but you cannot convince people by miracles if they are not ready to understand them.

Next, They started the Free Catholic Church, in which the priests and bishops could be married and have a family. Most of the priests were clairvoyant and healers, and when they talked you would see a Mahatma standing behind them and great globs of light fell from their lips when they spoke. It was exactly like the Roman Catholics, except they preached about the Mahatmas and it was completely occult. They had all the images of the Catholic Church: the altar, the holy water, everything, except they did not take confession and there was no allegiance to the Pope.

It was a form of the Church which took in the whole philosophy of metaphysics. But it also failed because only a handful of people will go to that sort of thing, because they feel it's not Catholic and it's not Protestant and they're afraid of it.

Then Agni Yoga came into being because of these failures. It was never taught in public until 1947. Up to that time it was a closed order, but in 1953 the whole movement began opening up and now there are other teachers in Europe. At first we were never allowed to say the things in class that we do now and if you notice, through the years we are allowed to give out more and more information so it's becoming more and more open all the time.

My Guru, Nicholas Roerich, was the first Teacher of Agni Yoga. It was a closed order of twenty-five people until 1936. It was always a closed circle. I knew some of the people but not all, as it wasn't necessary. Each one had their own work to do.

In 1947, I began to teach. I was the first teacher to be sent out from the Brotherhood in about a hundred years, because every hundred years the Teaching is given out and then it's withdrawn. This is done in cycles to coincide with certain dates and events. Now it will no longer be withdrawn because we are in the New Age.

As you know, September 17, 1936 at 9:15 P.M. was one of the important dates. That was the end of Kali Yuga and the beginning of Satya Yuga. Kali is the Sanskrit word meaning the "iron age" or "the age of materialism," and Satya means "light" or "illumination." The prophesy of the pyramids ran out on that date and many people thought it was going to be the end of the world, but it was only the end of a cycle.

The Hierarchy tells us, "We send you the people and you make no attempt to invite people or entice them to come or encourage them in any way. If they come you give them what they need and do it on their level." It's the idea of making the Teaching available for all who seek it. Once the door has been opened it can never be closed for any individual, no matter how obnoxious they become. That is a set rule of the esoteric order.

Agni Yoga was brought out as part of the whole plan of Theosophy. It's just another form of it; there is no real difference. Many times people argue that one was taken from the other, but it matters not, because there are many paths and they all lead to the sunlit snows. If this doesn't work out, another form of the Teaching will be brought out. There is this about Agni Yoga: it is never going to be for mass consumption or masses of people. The Teachings say, "Do not count the followers in the thousands, they exist in tens." It will never be given out in public. It will always be semiprivate, in the homes of people who have dedicated their homes for this particular study. Even in the New Age it will not be given out publicly. This is why the books we study are never advertised.

Many people have asked me about Masters and advertisements that are in the paper. This is one of the things to remember: there is no fee or price for esoteric study. If there is and you have to sign a contract and you are to get a diploma, this is nonsense. It doesn't work that way. An esoteric teaching can only be given out of love. It is never sold. You cannot buy it like meat and potatoes in the market, and that's how you know the difference. It is unfortunate that in Europe and America many people want to pay a fee to study with an organization and in some of the organizations you will learn many beneficial things, but you are not getting an esoteric teaching, and you never will. If a work is signed by Mahatma so and so, beware! Because no Mahatma will ever sign their name or ever tell you they are a Mahatma. Even if a Mahatma is working with a group of people and it is discovered that he is a Mahatma, he will disappear and completely vanish from the group.

3. The Mother of Agni Yoga is Madame Roerich. They also call her the White Tara. Tara means "female Mahatma." Many of the women in Agni Yoga are attuned to her and by reading everything you can find on the White Tara and Madame Roerich, you will come into a very close relationship with her.

4. I have a student in Montreal who said to me, "I have been having a class for about two years and I'm the only person in it." I said, "That's fine." She said, "I'm going to Vancouver. What shall I do?" I said, "The same thing."

A disciple of mine out in San Francisco had a class every Tuesday and Thursday evening for three years in which he would read from the Teaching and did his meditation and gradually at the end of that time the people began to come, in ones and twos and threes until now (1969) there are thirty-six students; very wonderful people who are doing wonderful things with the Teaching and applying it to their daily life.

5. Many people are intrigued by the phenomena in Agni Yoga. True, there is a great deal of phenomena but we discourage it because you should know the ethics and live for that. But, phenomena does happen and as you sensitize yourself these are proofs so that you have something to hang onto and can say, "I have experienced this and I know it." Many times people who are attracted to phenomena will never go any further. Clairvoyance and clairaudience are charming things and you can utilize them but it's not the end. It's only the beginning. The end is the idea of Cosmic Consciousness.

Swami used to explain it this way: here is the road straight ahead, and here are the little side roads of clairaudience and clairvoyance and all these things of phenomena. Now, you can get off on one of these side roads and get stuck there. It's alright to go off and investigate and then come back and go on down the straight road, but if you get stuck on a side street it may take another lifetime or two or three to come back. You must remember that the ultimate end is God Consciousness.

6. The whole principle of Yoga is that you yourself are working directly with divine wisdom and no intermediary is standing between you and God.

7. Agni Yoga is a game of truth and how to play it, but you must be honest with yourself. For instance, if you do something wrong, admit it. Say, "I made a mistake."

To illustrate this I often use the example of the glass. When you drop a water glass because you're not paying attention, what is your first reaction? You say, "The glass slipped out of my hand." This is dishonest thinking, when actually because of your carelessness or awkwardness you dropped it. The glass is an inanimate object. It can't move. But this is the way we lie to ourselves. We must be absolutely honest with ourselves and everyone else.

You must tell the truth but not harshly. When a lady comes up to you and says, "How do you like my new hat?" and it's really awful, say, "It's a pretty color"—if it is. Try to find something constructive to say about it and yet not lie. If someone comes and asks you, "What is wrong with me?" it is your duty to tell them. Whether they can take it or not is another thing. If they don't ask you, it's none of your business. When someone comes and asks, "What am I doing that irritates people?" you are actually doing them a favor by telling them.

There was a young chap I knew when I was going to Yale who had the faculty of putting his finger right on the sore spot. If you had a habit of one kind or another, he would tell you about it. Well, of course he had no friends and everyone laughed at him.

He was a very fine student and a wonderful man. He told me many things that were wrong with me. I said, "Anytime you see me doing anything irritating or anytime you see me acquiring a bad habit, tell me. I appreciate it."

Many years later I met him in New York and he said, "You know, R., I don't understand you. I've been nasty to many people including you but you've always been kind to me. You're the only friend I've ever had."

I said, "No, you may think you have been nasty to me, but you have taught me many wonderful things and in my gratitude I will give you my friendship for the rest of my life."

If we can work with this thing of truth, we can help one another and do it in a constructive way. So if someone comes and asks you if they have been doing something irritating, tell them. At least you have been a friend and have helped them.

Books of the Teaching

8. The books of Agni Yoga are never advertised. They are: *Leaves of Morya's Garden I (The Call); Leaves of Morya's Garden II (Illumination); Community; Agni Yoga; Infinity I; Infinity II: Hierarchy; Heart; Fiery World I; Fiery World II; Fiery World III; Aum; Brotherhood; Letters of Helena Roerich, Vol. I and II,* published by Agni Yoga Society, Inc., 319 West 107th Street, New York, New York.

The Letters of Helena Roerich are a compilation of letters written to the Guru, Nicholas Roerich, and answered by his wife. This is the first time the relationship between Guru and disciple has become open to the public. As a rule this is a very secret relationship, but these books have been published so that people might see the questions asked by the disciple and answered by the Guru.

You will never hear of these books unless it's by word of mouth. Certain bookstores handle them, but they only make about 20% profit while other books are marked up 40 to 50%. The idea is that when people are ready to hear about Agni Yoga they are sent. There is no accident; it all comes about by a great and beautiful design.

All occult books should be purchased. Never loan an occult book. There was a man who hitch-hiked all the way from San Francisco to study with me. He had very little money so I thought it would be a nice thing to do to give him a set of the books. So I talked to my sister in spirit and told her I would like to do this and she said, "No, don't. Let him go without lunch if necessary or sacrifice if necessary to buy one book. This he will read. Then give him the books but don't let him know where they came from." This is how we handled it.

If you give the books they will never be read. This is true of any occult esoteric book. It will never be read unless the person seeks it out and buys it himself. You couldn't possibly get anything out of a loaned book of Agni Yoga on the first, second or third reading, but if a person is truly interested and goes to the trouble to buy the book himself, then he can reread and reread and suddenly it makes sense.

Many people on a first reading say the books don't make any sense, and then maybe a year or two later they say that's a tremendous book. Suddenly they have an understanding and it comes through reading and rereading and absorbing. You can only absorb so much at one time. So they say, repetition, repetition and study and then you've got it.

The best form of study is to take three books and each morning read one or two or three paragraphs from each book and at night read them again. The next morning read three new ones. By doing this you start the day with that wisdom and at night you read this again so that it becomes part of your whole consciousness. This is the esoteric way it's done, by repetition, until it becomes part of you.

There are forty different interpretations to every verse in the Teaching. As you read the books over and over you will get the interpretation that suits your consciousness at that moment. You pick up a book and read it as a brand new book each time. That is why you never get through reading an esoteric book, never! I've been reading *The Mahatma Letters* for thirty years and it's like picking it up for the first time every time I read it. Many things are familiar, but when you break it down, like the letter on God, we spent four hours and only got halfway through it and it's only seven or eight pages long.

In your own study of the Teaching you should start with page one and proceed on through, but in a class you can open any book anywhere and what you read will be absolutely right for the situation. We never prepare for a class. If you prepare this is your ego saying, I'm going to read this for the benefit of the class when it may not be what they need at all. Invariably, it will be useless but when you pick a page at random people will come to you afterwards and say, "What you said tonight was personally directed to me, wasn't it?" Actually it was the Mahatmas who directed it because they knew what that person needed and wanted.

In reading the books of the Teaching, when They speak of Our or We, this refers to the Hierarchy. There is a beautiful passage in one of the books which says, "Give Us your anger, give Us your hatred, give Us your prejudice, give Us your greed, give Us all of these things and don't ask for them back." All words in the books that are capitalized refer to the Hierarchy. When you see "teacher" written with a small "t" it means the guru. This is a hard and fast rule.

9. Everything in the Teaching applies to life. Many times when you are faced with a difficult decision and there is no one around to help you, ask for help and then open one of the books of the Teaching and you'll get it. There it will be. It's happened over and over and I know of many people who have tried it and the right answer comes at the first moment.

I remember when I was in San Francisco. I had been there a year and if at the end of a year your mission is not accomplished you can leave, so I was dying to leave and it was just a year to the day and I said, "Good, I can go to L.A. and get out of San Francisco." I opened the book and it said, "We do not expect our messenger to fly the moment the year is up." I said, "Okay," and stayed another year and a half. It's amazing how this works. It's a very comforting thing to know.

10. Formerly in Tibet if a monk lost an argument he was confined to the Library for three days. He was sent there to read up on his subject so that next time he would know more than his opponent. Many times people will take a point and argue this point, and then they go beyond that and they don't know the next step and they bluff it.

I'll never forget a very amusing thing that happened in California. There was a lady who had a fabulous IQ and she would quote a certain book, page, and chapter and it was very impressive. One day she made the mistake of quoting something that I had memorized and it wasn't right at all. I told her about this and she said, "Well, it's very impressive anyway."

So many people read the books of the Teaching in hopes of getting this intellectually. This a thing of ego. They want to get it on their terms, in their way, without responsibility. The Teaching is a tremendous responsibility. This is true of any Teaching, and the moment we enter onto that path it's our responsibility—ethically, morally and in every way. Many people don't want to change and so they read these books and quote these beautiful things.

As the Teaching says, "When you give an old overcoat away with a tear, you haven't given anything." The important thing is service. In other words, if Joe Doaks' house burns down and you go to him and say, "Joe Doaks, I'm terribly sorry your house burned down," you are being dishonest, because you're not sorry. What this means is you're damn glad your house didn't burn down. If you are really sincere you will go to Joe Doaks and say, "Let me help you build your new house. Let me help you in any way, shape or form." And when you actually do it, then you are functioning karmically. This is an action. The other is lip service and has no value whatsoever. To me sympathy is a dirty word. Action is the thing.

Teaching of Living Ethics

11. Many people have the idea that the Mahatma will come privately and teach them. Many times people have come to me and

said, "Now we would like to come and study exclusively, privately."
I say, "I'm very sorry, but I don't work that way because the idea is
that of diversified people working together. This Teaching is not
exclusive. It's for the rich, the nobility, the poor, the famous, the
infamous, anyone who comes. It's available to anyone." The moment
you become exclusive about it you lose your contact with the
Hierarchy.

It's the idea that each student must develop himself or herself by
meditation, by study, by striving, and the more you strive and the
more you study, the more you will get. The Teacher can only open
the door, point the way and answer questions. The development is up
to the individual and you can't make a person do anything. They have
to do it on their own.

The more diversified the people in the group the greater the
magnetism and the better it is. If it's exclusive it's no good.

12. The natural thing for all people to have is a great
consciousness, and to live in truth and beauty, and it's a violation of
that right when you don't. This is your heritage, but unless you have
the zeal to make this come about, it will not come about, because the
Hierarchy does not force anything on anyone. They believe absolutely
in free will. This is why many times people never hear of any
Teaching whatsoever. It's not their destiny. It's not their karma.

Someone said the other day, "Suppose I had never heard of the
work." "But," I said, "you did, because you have earned the right.
You brought it to you by your development. You earned it in a former
life." Other people who are not ready for it have to come back again
and again to work it out. When you pick up a book or go to a movie
or a play there is always a message there, but how many people listen
to it?

13. How much should we tell about the Teaching? Many times
by opening the door too wide and telling too much we frighten people
away. In our zeal to share something wonderful we forget it's not the
right time. Let them ask but don't give more than they ask for.

One time Vivekananda was with a group of Holy Men and this
man came up to them and said, "Tell me about Shambhala. Tell me
about the Mahatmas." Vivekananda said, "I know of no such thing."
Later the Brothers said, "Why did you lie to this man?" And he said,
"This man did not ask out of purity of heart, but only out of
curiosity; therefore, cast not your pearls before swine or they will
turn and rend you."

Questions are good but curiosity is not. The Teaching is not just
a philosophy that you talk about, but it is a way of living twenty-four
hours a day and if you don't apply it you're not functioning and it

becomes a useless thing. Ask the people who approach you with questions, "What do you think about reincarnation?" and if they say, "There's nothing to it," walk away because you're just wasting your time. If they say, "I believe there's something to it," then next time you see them talk to them about maya and karma. But if they say, "When you're dead you're dead," walk off because all the talk in the world will not convince them.

There is a beautiful saying in the Brotherhood, and I quote Master Hilarion, "We wear the white robe of immortality which we must keep spotless not in fear of dirtying the robe but in fear for the people who throw mud upon it, that it will spatter back upon the thrower." This is the shield of protection for the people who attack the Teaching and thereby come under the law of karma which will react tenfold.

This you must remember: you are representative of the Hierarchy and you must protect that privilege. You shouldn't have anger or anguish, but you can be indignant. Like this woman who came to class one evening and began to criticize my Guru and I said, "You have a perfect right to criticize anyone you want in your own home or on the street, but not in my house, and I must ask you to leave." I had to be indignant. I was also doing her a favor because she was throwing mud on my Guru, not that He would mind, but the responsibility of what she was doing would come back to her tenfold.

14. The Teachings continually tell you, do not believe it because I have said it. Do not believe it because some sage has said it, or was inspired or thought he was inspired. Do not believe it because you have read it, but believe it when you know it in your own heart.

Question everything but never doubt, because when you doubt the door is closed forever. I was talking to some people in England and they were saying they can see the little people. It's quite common for many people in Ireland and Scotland to see them. They said, "Why is it so difficult for Americans to see them?" I said, "It's simple, because they don't believe and when they say it doesn't exist, it doesn't for them." If you say, "I believe anything can happen," it will. There is a very thin line between doubting and questioning and when you say, "I question," you are asking to know more, but when you say, "I doubt it," you have closed the door and whatever it is you doubt is impossible for you to experience.

15. Your subconscious mind from all your past lives can be compared to a great pot on the stove. In this pot are potato peels and apple peels and cores and everything else, and as that boils the garbage comes to the top and flows out and over. When this happens, you are eliminating all the garbage from your heart, all the ugly thoughts, the

negative thoughts, and destructive things. This is why the beautiful speech of Buddha, "All about you is great light and great joy. All you have to do is reach out and touch it and it is beyond the wildest dreams of man."

You never lose anything you have attained, never! All knowledge, every experience you have gone through—you have gained from it, haven't you? So what you do is keep adding lifetime after lifetime of wisdom, knowledge, patience, love and understanding, and you never lose it. You may stand still in your development for a lifetime or two, but you do not lose what you have up to that point. There is no retrogression. It does not exist. There's only progression.

Any person who attends a class of esoteric teaching for two years has earned the right for discipleship. That doesn't mean you are going to be accepted but you have earned the right. When you come to the point of reaching discipleship, most of your karma is gone; let's say ninety percent of it. The rest of it the teacher takes on and throws it off in his aura, so that you start with a clean slate from all your past lives. This is why they call it the "unseen gift." Of course, you can make more karma from then on, but by doing good for humanity and keeping it a secret you can keep that karma balanced out and be as free of karma as you were at initiation. It's doing a whole lot in a short space of time, but you can do it if you take the Teaching and apply it in your life. If you come to class and sit there and don't take it into your life and work with it, you're not doing anything.

The very fact that you are drawn to a group of people and will work and devote your life to that means you've earned it and you've put it into practice. As the Hierarchy says, "Give us your anger. Give us your fear. Give us all the ugly things that you have about you and we will take them and destroy them." But naturally you must give something in return.

Every person knows why they don't make progress after becoming a disciple. All you have to say is, "What am I doing wrong?" and you will get the answer very fast. Of course, then the person has to do something about it.

I will never forget this lovely, charming, beautifully educated woman who had traveled all over the world, and one night in class I said that Christ was a Jew, which was true. She said, "I can't accept that." And do you know for years she sent me pictures of Christ as an Aryan, with blue eyes and blond hair which was ridiculous as he was a Jew. Here was a person with a fine mind but full of blocks, and if a person is blocked they are not going to face the truth. It's the idea of "don't convince me with facts, my mind is made up."

I've been healing since I was sixteen years old and I'm sixty now. I've got thirty-three disciples and I'm lucky to have that many. [When this was published fifteen years later, there were between 95-100 disciples.] Many disciples in this life were disciples in a former life. Do not count it in thousands, it exists in tens.

16. Before 1936, it was as Helena Roerich said in her letters, "...it is inadmissable to entrust something holy to paper which passes through so many hands because much would be destroyed or harmfully interpreted." In great antiquity the Teaching of Light was transmitted orally or in veiled symbols. There was great goal–fitness and co–measurement in this. This is why Christ taught in parables, but then the Church took it all literally and made dogma of it and they lost the whole essence of it.

For instance, "Cast your bread upon the waters..." means the tenfold law of karma, and when He said, "Life everlasting," this is your reincarnation. Immortality means "without beginning and without end," but it's been distorted. It's only in the last ten years that people will use the word reincarnation and discuss it. Before that it was a dirty word.

Right now there are many of the hippies who are wearing the clothes and various trappings of the Indians. These kids are again interested in the mysticism that the Indians are steeped in, and they are really fine occultists. The Indians feel these people are the reincarnation of the old Indians come back to do their work.

The hippies out in Taos call themselves Warriors of the Rainbow, and they are. The Teaching often speaks about the rainbow. When you see a rainbow it means a great event has taken place somewhere in the world, and when you see a double rainbow, you really have something. It's a world event that has taken place in the consciousness of humanity. So, the rainbow has a very great significance. The Irish talk about the pot of gold at the end of the rainbow. This means the rainbow is the bridge between the mundane and Subtle Worlds and the bridge to the Hierarchy with the consciousness to travel astrally. In Tibet, when a falling star appears, this means a great Teacher has appeared on the Earth—a great soul has come to teach.

17. We were having this conversation about Agni Yoga with a doctor in Pennsylvania that we know when his brother came and sat listening. We were talking about karma and the law of cause and effect, etc., and suddenly he jumped up and said, "But you're too strict." I said, "No, we're not too strict. The law is the law and you must live by it. There can be no deviation. It must be all or nothing. You can't do it by giving 99½%, it has to be 100%." It's very difficult to surrender yourself 100%, because the old ego says, "I want to do it

my way." This is where the heart and devotion and goal-fitness come in.

Goal fitness means being completely honest and sincere and doing everything the right way, in a completely ethical way. To talk ethics means nothing, but when you live it and practice it then it means something because you're working with the cosmic law. Many people go to church and pray but they don't live it. You must live it twenty-four hours a day, not one hour a week; then you have goal-fitness. It's called goal-fitness because the goal is God Consciousness, and the only way to get there is to play the game of life. Agni Yoga is one way to play the game and it's as sharp as the razor's edge. It's not deviating to the right or left, but right straight down the middle. You're either following the path or you're not, so why kid yourself!

18. There is no retrogression. The one consoling fact is you cannot retrogress, but you can stand still for a whole lifetime. If you do nothing in this life, you do nothing in the Subtle World between lives.

Anyone can make a mistake. You may know all the cosmic laws, and yet go against them. If you do, you will have to pay the karma. But no one can take away the knowledge you already have. That you can never lose. It's forever and ever. As you go through life from lifetime to lifetime, you keep building this knowledge. If you want to sit and not use it, that is your choice, but you don't retrogress.

The fallen angel is the idea that people are working in ignorance. Nothing is bad. Everything is just an experience. As God is everything, how can you separate it? There is no separation. It's only lack of discrimination.

Once I asked the Swami Bodhinanda, "What is sin?" He said, "There is no such thing. The only sin is that people are not happy. They are not in their true place in life, walking in the Light. Whatever else is done by man is called by many names but it's still karma. It may be he has to go through that experience to learn something from it."

When finally man gets tired of living in ignorance, then he can do something about it and change that karma. It's like the man who was hitting his head with a hammer. Someone asked him, "What are you doing that for?" and he said, "Because it feels so good when I stop."

In the Bible it says, ". . . the sins of the father shall be visited on the third and fourth generation." This is karma. It means they will come back into that same family. Family relationships are always karmic. They may be good karma or bad, but you have some karma to work out with these people or you wouldn't be in that family.

So when you can say: "This is my karma, I have earned it from before and I will not bitch about it or complain;" and when you can say: "Give it to me and I will try to understand the situation;" and when you do, then you will no longer have disappointment or antagonism or any of these negative things. So you say, "Let me pay it off fast," and you will.

19. This is the thing we have all gone through and that is as you grow on this path, you find you are alone and then you find your fellow travelers, but they are few and far between. You find you no longer have anything in common with your old friends and it's a sad thing but there it is. You are growing and they are standing still and you can't take them with you because they won't come.

20. It used to be that a neophyte began study at the age of thirty, but this is no longer true. Now they begin at twelve and thirteen. In the New Age it's completely different.

21. In the Teaching They say, "We give you hints," and then it's up to the individual to work with them and experiment, because there are no two people alike either physically, mentally or spiritually. Each one is at a different level. Each one is approaching the Teaching in a different way, so when you are given a hint and you think it may be important, then you pursue it.

22. Oftentimes people in the Teaching seem to come to a plateau and stop and rest for awhile. You do not climb the mountain straight up without resting. You ascend plateau by plateau.

23. In the Teaching you find this happens: many times the people in the group will sit in the same place or near that location. I asked the Swami Bodhinanda one day why it was that when I come in to class I want my usual seat. He said, "When you are working with people on a spiritual basis, they will sit together by incarnation. The various people who have been Chinese will sit together. The Indians will sit together, the Egyptians, and so on and so forth. Now, without looking at the individual, you send an unspoken thought from your heart to theirs."

This is actually a great part of the Teaching, not what is said, but what is left unsaid. As you progress in your work and develop there will come a day when words will not be necessary. There will be a complete exchange of information from heart to heart without any spoken words. As people develop the use of the heart, they will be able to converse at any time and at any distance, after death, beyond it and then into the next life. Visualize your Guru sitting beside you in the car or plane. This is good practice in tuning in to your Guru, and learning how to engage in a heart to heart conversation.

24. One evening I was at a gathering with a group of my disciples. I met an old friend of mine who had been in the Russian Intelligence Agency. He was very sophisticated and had traveled all over the world. He was telling me, "You know we were trained that people have two faces. And do you know Mr. H., I observe a very interesting thing. You people have only one face. It's right there and you can read it."

This is very true. When you've been in the Teaching for awhile this duplicity falls away. Many times we have had people who came to the Teaching with the intention of using it for their own purposes, but it's bigger than they are and they end up by it using them.

25. The seven ways of caution: One of the great ways is discrimination in talking to people about the Teaching when they aren't ready for it. Many times in our enthusiasm we want to share something we have discovered with somebody else and they reject it. I've made this mistake myself. One time I had a lad who was on fire with the Teaching. His aura was simply amazing. We told him too much of the whole structure of the Hierarchy and he ran off. It was too much. He was frightened to death of the responsibility and he ran out the door and we never saw him again. Never tell too much. This is why they say never take this Teaching into the market place and try to sell it to passersby. They aren't ready.

This reminds me of the story of the man who carried this dog into the market place and he thought it was God. He said, "God, if you will allow me to do this all these people will see you and they will all change." So he put God on his shoulder and went into the market place and the people were repulsed. What they saw was a dog covered with ugly sores. People will only see what they are ready to see and what you see is not for everyone else.

26. In the Teaching it says, "...to drink the chalice of poison." This means the ugliness in the world, the hatred, the anger, the thing of nation against nation, blacks against whites—this is the chalice of poison. What They mean by drinking it: this means to go out and work to try to solve these problems. When you have peace within yourself you can give it to others. If you have turmoil within yourself, you give turmoil. If you have prejudices, you give that. So, if you can take all these things away from people, this is drinking the cup of poison.

Light is coming, but it is coming with great difficulty. People want to hang onto their old ways of doing things in the world, but we have to throw away the old ideas and get brand-new ones that will work better. This is where you find the gap between youth and older people.

Many highly evolved people are drinking this chalice of poison. I quote from the Teaching, "Many people play small and ugly roles in this life and very unhonored roles in order to accomplish this. . ." Principally this poison is the thoughts of people who have hatred. You go into a room where there is hatred and it hits you like a knife. Where there is peace and love you feel that too, and it's a very good feeling.

27. The Teaching says, "It is better to ride in one's own canoe even if it has holes, than to ride in another's ship." This means this is like riding somebody else's coattails, or like someone who picks your brain and passes off the information as his own, or when you blame someone else for your mistakes. Like the people who take credit for something that someone else has developed and passes it off as their own idea. It's also taking credit away from another individual.

The great trick of esoteric occultism is always give credit where credit it due. Many people want to take the information they have and hand it out as their own. This is one area in which my Guru instructed me very carefully; whenever anyone tells you anything always quote them as the source of your information. This is very important.

Yogis

28. When you as a yogi have allied yourself with the Brotherhood, you are helped. I quote from the Teaching, "Not only is a yogi a blessing to his family, but to his country, to the planet, to the planetary system and all people connected with him or her, including the people with whom you come in daily contact." This is part of the unseen gift that is given and bestowed on a yogi.

Yoga means "Union with God," and this is a tremendous power for good and it affects the lives of all people who come in contact with it. It's called the philosopher's stone and is often symbolized by a great diamond, the idea being that the diamond is pure crystal, beautifully cut, absolutely clean and pure, has great strength and cannot be destroyed.

29. In the Teaching it speaks of movability of consciousness. This means that wherever a yogi or yogini goes, this is home; no matter what country or people. You do not take your culture with

you, you adapt and adjust to their customs and culture. This makes you very pliable in your thinking and you see things from their perspective. One of the very great Truths in your approach to people is "not by my God but by thy God." You should try to see their form of God through their eyes, because if you approach them with your idea of God, then you are forcing your philosophy on them and this is forbidden.

30. A very good student of Yoga is one who applies everything in the book to himself. When you listen and you say, "I might be operating like this," this is excellent. But the student who says, "Oh no, this is beyond me, I've got it made, I don't have to worry," this is dangerous. He's really stepping on thin ice.

31. Some people think they are going to be great yogis or yoginis in two or three weeks. There's a lot of phony businesses where you can get a quick course in yoga and a diploma for a few hundred dollars.

One day two ladies came to dear old Swami Bodhinanda who was just a tremendous man. His path was Bhakti, *[The yoga of love]*. He was very sincere and humble, beautifully eductated, taught Sanskrit, and spoke beautiful English. These ladies said to him, "We'd like to become great yoginis." He said, "I boo to you." He never could say "bow" very well. They said, "Now, how long is this going to take?" He said, "Well Mesdames, I have been studying to be a yogi for seventy-two years." So they said, "If you aren't a yogi in seventy-two years, we don't want you. You can't know very much. We can go down to 57th Street and for two hundred dollars we can get a gold certificate that says we are a yogini." He said, "Mesdames, I boo to you."

32. As I have stated before there are less than one hundred Mahatmas and not everyone is destined to achieve Mahatmaship, not even in the seventh race of the seventh round. So I have been asked what then is the highest achievement we can attain here on Earth.

To become an Adept is a great achievement. To become a fine householder is another wonderful thing. An Adept is very close to Mahatmaship and a good householder is quite an accomplishment.

To be a yogi in the true sense of the word is also quite an accomplishment, for this is wisdom. This is the idea that you are one with the Microcosm and Macrocosm; or stated another way, you, Nature, God and Cosmos are one.

It would be very nice to be a Mahatma, but I am content to be what I am and try to make this a better world. We should not be concerned with ourselves or our future but think only of how we can serve. The very fact that you aspire to be a Mahatma will defeat your purpose. We should be desireless and devote our life to service for humanity.

We are here for one purpose and that is to make this a better world. We may not be able to do it but our children are going to do it. So you ask yourself, what can you do to help the children? How can you open doors for them? When people come to me and say, "I don't know what to do with my life," I tell them, "Be a teacher. You can open doors for the child that even their father and mother cannot open; doors they never dreamed existed."

In Texas there is a school conceived by the Hierarchy and operated under the direction of Morya. Here children from two to five are taught how to read in new ways. Mathematics are taught with colored rods. They are taught English and Spanish. They are taught meditation.

The children are completely integrated. There are black and white and Chinese and there is no prejudice in the minds of these children. They don't know it. They are taught that all children can work and play together.

Now, when a child has been exposed to this kind of environment up to the time they are seven years of age, they are free. They are not going to get all mixed up in later years. These children will in a few short years grow up to be the leaders of tomorrow and herein lies our hope for making this a better world.

33. It is not good for yogis to give their eyes or heart or various organs to medical science because this will damage the subtle body, and when you come back in the next life there will be a weakness in that area. It's part of the seed of the spirit. Like J.V. who lost her eyesight in a fire in a previous life and this time she has had great difficulty with her eyes. She has had four corneal transplants and they won't hold.

It takes several lifetimes to get over something like this. You come in with all this weakness. In one of my incarnations in France I was paralyzed, and this is something I always have to watch very carefully, to keep moving and exercise. That was a long time ago and I've had several incarnations since then.

Your body is a shell which you leave behind, but your astral (or subtle) body still carries that scar and when the astral body dissolves, that scar is still part of your subconscious memory, which you carry into the next life. This memory bank is in that part of the brain (the cerebellum) that is 70% unused. For instance, if you have a terrible fear of water, it's because you have drowned in a past life, but if you can recall the memory of it, that fear will go away.

Also, it's not good to give blood to someone else unless it's to someone of the same consciousness, because through yoga your alchemy has changed your blood chemistry, and if you put that blood into someone of a lower consciousness, it will shock them and do a lot of damage. Their consciousness lifts and they are not ready for it. On the other hand, if you accept blood from someone who is not as developed and is not working consciously, it will affect your whole system.

On death, cremation is the ideal thing, to consume the body as quickly as possible, but not to dissect the body or take out the eyes. It's a very nice idea to offer your body for science and there are hundreds of people who will do this but that's up to them. When you are in a Teaching, you know better and you won't do it.

Maitreya

34. The Buddha is always shown with one foot up in the lotus position and one foot down, symbolizing the prophesy of the coming of the Maitreya. The Maitreya [statue of] is always standing, meaning that he will walk on Earth. The Maitreya is here and has been seen since 1955, but as far as I know He has not yet spoken to any group. Evidently we are not ready to hear what He has to say. As we develop and work toward God Consciousness, this will take place.

The Maitreya has been prophesied for some eight thousand years as the Avatar who will come and bring a new Teaching to the world. And those people who are studying and working with this Teaching have been sent at this particular time to work with the Maitreya and prepare the way for His coming. On the cover of the Agni Yoga books there is a symbol in Tibetan which means, "The Coming of Lord Maitreya."

There is an interesting story told to me by a very charming English couple who came to one of my classes as students. He was an engineer and traveled all over the world. He was coming back to San Francisco from one of his trips to Australia but stopped off in India enroute. At the New Delhi airport he had about four hours to wait, so he said, "Shall I stay here and wait or go into town?" So he decided to hire a horse and buggy—called a "tonga"—and go into town. He had just paid the driver when this man in a yellow robe walked up and called him by name and said, "Do you remember me?" and he said, "Yes, you were the abbot in Cambodia that I asked about the Maitreya. I asked you when is He coming and where will He appear?"

The abbot said, "Yes, that is correct, and do you remember that when you asked those questions I couldn't tell you but I promised to tell you at another time? I knew you were coming here today and I came to intercept you and tell you that He will appear in 1965 in San Francisco."

So my student made the rest of his journey and came on to visit his friends in San Francisco and there on the table were the Agni Yoga books. He picked one up and said, "My God, where did you get these?" and they said, "We're studying this philosophy." He said, "Do you know what you are studying?" and they said, "Well, we think we do." He said, "Do you know about the Maitreya?" and they said, "Yes," and then he told them this story.

About 1953 I was sent to San Francisco on a mission. I was not told what I was to do or what the mission was. They said, "You can go on this mission if you choose but you must remain there for at least a year." So I went, but I had no idea that this was a preparation for the Maitreya.

The work was rejected. We couldn't get enough people interested long enough. They wanted phenomena. So, after two and a half years we were told to go to Los Angeles, which we did and then we were told to come back to New York.

But while we were in Los Angeles, five of us were having a meditation one day at the Vedanta Center under the pepper tree where the parking lot is now. One of the people touched me and we looked and there He was, but only four of the five saw Him. He performed a special little thing and we all wrote it down and got it exactly right. It was a most beautiful and wonderful thing to see.

I would say He looks between thirty-four and thirty-six years old. He has a very clear complexion and a reddish beard and reddish hair—almost titian. His eyes are extremely green, like green grapes. He was in a white robe and wore open sandals that laced like old Roman sandals, but each lace was of a different color. There was a sort of rope around his waist, very much like the monks wear. We saw him in a physical form.

Since then He has appeared to various people—about three times here in New York. One night at B.M.'s in New York, we were looking at a film of Roerich's paintings. We had just finished and the lights came on and five people saw Him. He was also seen in northern Michigan and over on Staten Island, and each time there have been five people present. It seems five is a very important number. Whenever you have five, seven or twelve people present in a meeting, not counting the leader, you have a perfect number.

The Maitreya appeared during the meditation at eleven o'clock in the morning of November 22, on the day we put the cornerstone in place and dedicated the Ashram (at Smithville Flats, New York). In the cornerstone there is the hand, the foot, the pillar and arch and the Roerich Pact and Banner of Peace symbol. There is a prophesy as Christ said, "When these symbols appear on the cornerstone, there will be seven stars appear above this temple and this will mean that the New Age is founded and at work." As far as I know this is the first time these symbols have been laid in any cornerstone at any place on this planet. This is why the Ashram is a magnet and why we receive all these powerful energies.

35. This is the first time an Avatar has come from outside our solar system. This is why the New Age is such a tremendous thing.

Only the highest kind of unity will create a medium for the Maitreya to manifest. When you transcend all the garbage that is within you and the pure form of God that is within you comes out, then you are functioning in this unity. When any group is in perfect harmony with one another, in trust and faith and love, He will manifest by using the atoms of your various bodies to create His own atoms and in doing so He will lift up your energies. He will materialize and teach us just as I sit here and teach and then He will dematerialize again. He is not only going to come to students of Agni Yoga but He will come to all groups where the people are working together for Light.

It must be done that way because if He came as an ordinary man what would they do to Him? The same thing they did to Christ and Buddha. So this is His protection.

Buddha taught release from the wheel of karma and He was not accepted. After that Christ came to teach the pure simple message of love. What happened? The Inquisition in Spain and the terrible wars fought under the name of God. This is not love. Now the Maitreya is coming to teach through cosmic law and divine wisdom; to teach people not to kill one another just because they disagree. The key is diversified people working together; all the different nationalities, all the different ideas, all the different religions, by joining hands and working together through the media of love and understanding and wisdom. It has to come through the opening up and inspiring of people and through the intellect. It has to be a special wisdom. As they say in the East, "Joy is a special wisdom."

36. In the Teaching they speak of the double Avatar. This is the Maitreya and Rigden Jeppo. They are one and the same. One day I was talking to Norbu, the brother of the Dalai Lama at the Museum of Natural History, and I said, "I would like very much to have a tanka of Shambhala." And he said, "Shambhala? You know of Shambhala?"

I said, "Yes, Roerich wrote a book on it. I have it in my library." He said, "In Tibet only the high lamas know of Shambhala."

We continued to talk and he brought out a banner and I said, "That's not the one I'm looking for." He said, "Which banner are you looking for?" I said, "Rigden Jeppo." His face fell open and he said, "You know that name?" I said, "Yes, very well." He said, "You know the meaning of it?" I said, "Yes, He and the Lord Maitreya are one." He said, "My God!" I said, "This is what Roerich teaches his students. He's a great esoteric Guru." And he said, "He certainly is."

37. The coming of the Maitreya is called the second coming of Christ by the Christians. The Buddhists call it the second coming of Buddha. The Mohammedans call it the second coming of Allah. The Jews call it the second coming of Moses, but it isn't any of these. It's a new Avatar coming with this whole new idea of God Consciousness in everything. His message has to be bigger than our present concepts because we are not living together in peace. We're killing each other for no reason at all, but if we understand one another then we can begin to move.

The Maitreya will be teaching on other planets in our solar system as well, but they will not need the same teaching as we do. Earth is the third lowest in the planetary scale. Saturn is the lowest, then Mars and then Earth. All the others are higher than we are. Thank God!

This simple thing of loving each other is a beautiful thing to see. For instance, in one of the groups in California, there are eight disciples and this is a perfect example of the kind of love that can exist between people. You can touch it, it's so beautiful. There is complete harmony, complete trust; it's a complete brotherhood, no bickering or fault finding or complaining.

As the Teachings say, "We are brothers and sisters of spirit." Your true family is not your personal family, but as Christ said, "He who gives up mothers and fathers and brothers and sisters will have even more mothers and fathers and brothers and sisters, and he who gives up houses will have even more houses." Your blood relation is a karmic thing and your spiritual relation is a thing you have earned. Agni Yoga is actually the teaching of Shambhala and many times disciples are referred to as princes and princesses of Shambhala of spirit. This is the true royalty of consciousness and spirit. As Buddha said, "Guard well your tongues, that they be palace doors, a king within tranquil and fair and courteous be all words from which that presence went."

Hierarchy

38. When you have the link with Hierarchy, it's an endless course of learning, and you develop and develop and develop and never stop. It's like taking a course in college that never ends, yet you do it from lifetime to lifetime, and once you are conscious of this you can really make it a better world for humanity. People like Frank Lloyd Wright, and Nikola Tesla—who left 1,500 inventions to help people—and George Washington Carver and many others were brought in and given special tasks to do to help make life a little easier for humanity on this Earth.

True, our government is a hierarchy, our family is a hierarchy, the Church is a hierarchy but the Hierarchy we are speaking of is the Mahatmas or Masters as they are sometimes called. They work on both the subtle plane and in the mundane world and their job is to make this a better world. I quote from the Teaching, "We use plane tickets, boat tickets, train tickets and We walk among men." They are in governments; they are in art, science, music, in everything of a nature that lifts the consciousness of people. That's their whole purpose. They are an inspiration to all mankind.

Up until 1935 only two Mahatmas were created every one hundred years. There are less than one hundred Mahatmas in our solar system. The number remains fixed and as new Mahatmas ascend, two become Dhyan Choans, and two Dhyans become Lords of the planet and so on. So this is the way it operates. When you reach a certain stage of development you are told the exact number of Mahatmas. This is a known number but you can only know it when you are told; you then take this number to your Guru, and if it is correct, this is your proof that you have received your first message from your Mahatma. But the number has to be correct.

This is like trying to find the Dalai Lama. When they find a child they believe to be the reincarnation of the Dalai Lama, five hundred objects are place on the floor before Him. Some are His from a past life and some are other people's, and He is asked to choose those that belonged to Him. If He makes one mistake, they won't accept Him.

When they were looking for the present Dalai Lama, the abbot of this monastery disguised himself as a servant so he could go out into the kitchen and talk to this little three-year-old child. It was winter and the abbot was heavily robed and wore a high collar and tunic. As he held the little boy in his lap the child said, "You're wearing my necklace. Give it back." It was true, he was wearing the necklace under all this cloth. This is how they found the Dalai Lama.

Then in the big test there was an umbrella. The child said, "That's mine." And they said, "No, this is an error." But he said, "No, it was given to me in my former life and I gave it to the abbot." When the abbot he had mentioned was questioned, the story was found to be absolutely true.

39. Each person has an individual covenant with the Hierarchy, between your consciousness and that of the Hierarchy. This is why you must be absolutely on your own and free. The majority of people work through the churches which is another medium entirely. They put the responsibility on the Rabbi, the Priest, or the Minister, but the responsibility is yours and not theirs.

In the first place all the churches and temples were ever meant for was meditation. Each man is individually responsible to the laws of karma or Nature or whatever you want to call it, but when the Priests and Ministers and Rabbis began to take over, all this changed. They said Christ died for your sins, so you can go ahead and do anything you want. It's a very light-minded method of taking the responsibility away from people.

With this they took the covenants away as well, but we are responsible, every one of us directly, and we can't put the blame on anyone else or pass the buck. If we do something that's wrong, it's wrong and therefore we must pay for it, tenfold, and ignorance of the law is no excuse. It's just like in physical laws, ignorance is no excuse.

If the law of karma and reincarnation were taught in the schools and churches, believe me, there would be no more theft or murder or rape or wars, because everyone would know they are directly responsible for their actions, good or bad, and they must pay for them. If this were brought into the lives of children, we wouldn't have all this difficulty we're in now, but these things are political for the purpose of domineering the other individual.

This is what we mean when we say the soul must be absolutely free. You must never domineer another soul or another consciousness in any way, shape or form. You help them, yes; not by your God, but by their God, by their standards. Don't try to change them to your way of thinking, because theirs is a very individual matter. It's a covenant between them and their consciousness, a very sacred thing, and must never be interfered with in any way, shape or form, or threat. When people threaten you with excommunication or things like that, don't believe it—it's impossible. No human being can excommunicate you from God. You are one with it. They do it to try to dominate you, and this is completely wrong.

40. The oldest Mahatma is called Jupiter, the Ancient One. He is one of the early Mahatmas who came from the planet Jupiter which is spiritually the highest and most important planet in our planetary system. He's Indian. He's in Shambhala.

As Earth is a school, so each man and woman has to walk the path on Earth, and through their development has to reach Mahatmaship. In this way Roerich became a Mahatma and Madame Roerich a Tara. King Akbar became Morya. This was the first King Akbar of India who brought to a very primitive people all the great art, all the great culture, all the great poetry from Iran and Turkey and all over the world. Through beauty and education he actually created the whole Indian empire. The Ajanta caves and all of these things are the result of Akbar.

I have been asked many times, "What is the difference between a Mahatma and Buddha?" Let me put it this way; a Mahatma is the superintendent and Buddha is the president. Buddha means complete enlightenment.

In the Hierarchy of Light you begin with the Mahatmas and above them are the Dhyan Choans who help the Mahatmas with special decisions. Then there are the Kumaras who are the Lords of the planet and beyond them you have the four Lords of Karma. Jesus is the head of the Ashram of the Mahatmas in Shambhala. Rigden Jeppo is the King or Ruler of Shambhala.

These men and women who devote their lives to this work are actually like guardian angels to the planet. For instance, Roerich was an archaeologist and anthropologist. He left 8,000 paintings, 28 books, the Pact and Banner of Peace. He was an attorney, a Russian Prince, and would have won the Nobel Peace Prize when war was declared. He founded the Roerich Foundations in London, Paris and New York, Philadelphia, Rome, Brussels, Antwerp and Latvia.

In New York, the Hierarchy gave the plan for the Master Institute. In it there was a very large, beautifully equipped theater. They taught rhythmics, sculpture, ballet, art, writing. His idea was to make this center a brain trust and bring together all the best minds of Europe in the fields of science and the arts, which he did, and then in 1932 there was a great deal of dissention and this scattered it to the winds.

41. Many times people will say, the Teachings are written by Morya. They are written by Morya. Actually, they are written by

practically the whole of Hierarchy. It is not the work of one man but the work of many people who are the bridge to the Hierarchy. They all contributed to each book. You can tell by the way it's written that Morya wrote it, but others who also wrote are Koot Hoomi, Hilarion, the Venetian Master, Serapis and Jupiter, who is one of the ancient ones, and the Lord Maitreya.

There is no separation in the way the Mahatmas work to help us. They are here to give us knowledge, to give us wisdom, to give us understanding. They combine their forces. For instance, Morya and Koot Hoomi work together very closely. They are almost inseparable. Many people who are under the ray of Koot Hoomi are also under Morya's ray. Wherever there is a need they are there.

It's like a tremendous computer and these are facts and that's why they call it Straight Knowledge. When you are attuned to this knowledge it is available to you for your development. There are no short cuts. Actually the Teaching is a form of programming on the IBM machine, only this is the Hierarchy machine. This is why on the cover of the books of the Teaching there is this little symbol which means the "Coming of the Lord Maitreya." This Teaching is the preparation for that coming. These are the instructions and rules on how to play the game of life. It's extremely simple and extremely direct.

42. An Avatar and an Arhat are the same thing. They come at specific times, when they are needed, like Buddha who came 2,500 years ago and Christ who came 2,000 years ago.

An Adept is one who is developing toward Mahatmaship and is usually between the sixth and seventh initiation. Their clairvoyance and clairaudience are opened and they are well on the way to Mahatmaship. George Washington, Ben Franklin, Jefferson and the one they called the Old Professor were all Mahatmas or Adepts.

We were in Philadelphia recently and saw the Declaration of Independence with all the signatures. Suddenly I could see all of these men sitting in this room making all of these revolutionary laws, and I was filled with the realization that if it weren't for them none of us would be here. They had the daring, the courage, the foresight to envision this new country, this New World, as it's called. The bigotry and all the old laws of the Old World were left behind. Something brand-new and clean and fresh had been formed here.

And as we continued our tour from the House of Representatives to the Senate chambers I had the feeling of the birth of this country. As you know, Philadelphia was the first capitol. The first bank still stands. Ben Franklin's School of Philosophy still stands. The trade unions, which were a secret order of the Brotherhood, still stand. All of these old buildings have been restored and to walk through them is like going back into the history of our country. It's an exciting experience.

The man who was always introduced as the Professor designed the flag, and this is on display in the Library of Congress along with his speeches. This man ate fruits and nuts and never drank or smoked and he was the one who offered all these fiery speeches.

When it was time to sign the Declaration of Independence, the men in the Continental Congress suddenly realized they could all be hung as traitors for what they were about to do, and there was a reluctance to sign. Suddenly, in the balcony (which was locked), a man rose and gave this fiery speech, which can still be found in the Library of Congress. He spoke about freedom of religion, freedom of country, about independence, and when he had finished, they all rushed forward to sign. They turned to thank him but he was gone. The guards at the door said no one had entered and no one had left. He was a Mahatma. They needed that fire at that moment.

43. Your chosen ideal [chosen image] is one of the Avatars such as: Jesus, Moses, Buddha, Mohammed. A disciple is accepted by his chosen ideal or Mahatma at the time of the fourth initiation which is called Christos. This is the Greek word meaning Cosmic Consciousness. It happens to all initiates regardless of their race, color, creed or approach to the Teaching. This is the initiation of Isis and the veil is torn away after which the individual has the ability to see beyond into the fourth dimension and this is called Straight Knowledge. You do not see your chosen image, but you do see the whole thing of Isis which is the image of the Mother of the World and you have this whole experience while you're wide awake.

When Helena Roerich says, "The Teacher appears and the disciple is accepted," this means the Teacher appears after you have attended three times to the study of any form of Teaching. After you have attended three times in a row you attract the Mahatma or Teacher and They will then watch you as you develop and guide you and protect you and watch over you. You are the flowers in Their garden and They are the gardeners and They feed and shelter you and take care of you, but They do not become visible until after the fourth initiation.

Everyone is given this opportunity, but many people are asleep. For instance, if anyone has a great love for Christ or Buddha—a true devotion—they open that door with that devotion. Devotion is actually the whole power and motivation of one's spiritual development. When you can send that love, that Bhakti to a particular Avatar, then you have the key. As Roerich said in his book

Realm of Light, "You can't feel true love until your Teacher is in your heart."

44. The shield and the arrow: The arrow is a thought that goes out into space. If I send you a thought it is directed to you like an arrow. The idea of the shield is the protective shield of the Hierarchy. They say, "Give us your anger, your troubles, your irritation, and this shield of protection of the Hierarchy will be your armor."

The only thing that will penetrate that armor is doubt. Everyone of you is impregnable, but doubt is like a chink in your armor and when this happens you are lost because your armor has been pierced.

Take your difficulties to the Hierarchy and say, show me how to get out of them, teach me how, lead me. Give yourself to Them. Let Them do it and They will. You're asking for Their help and guidance, and this is the whole idea of working with wisdom. When you're working on that level, you are given wisdom and you use it. As they say in the Teaching and I quote, "When you are on the edge of the abyss, then help will come but only at the last moment." Otherwise we are asking the Hierarchy to do things for us we can do for ourselves. It's like sending God to the store for gingerale. Earlier I told you the story of the woman in San Francisco who left a beautiful white coat in her unlocked car. I said, "Do you think that is wise?" and she said, "Jesus will watch over it." This is a sacrilege. Anything we can do for ourselves we should do.

Then if there is a great need, if someone who is not in the Teaching is in great difficulty you may ask the Hierarchy how to help and guide them and you will be given direction and guidance. For your own problems, try to work it out, but if you can't then give it to the Hierarchy.

It's like the chisel and the hammer in the hands of the sculptor. The chisel is used to make this beautiful statue from a piece of marble and then the chisel says, didn't I create a beautiful masterpiece, but it was the sculptor with the hammer that did it. So always remember, you are the chisel and God is the sculptor with the hammer.

45. The very fact that you have a connection with the Hierarchy helps those around you. For instance, one of my disciples was in the army and he was more intellectual than athletic. He's the one who knows all the languages. So, when he was going through basic training he was taking the test of running with full pack and he failed miserably. He was frightened that he would have to go through the whole basic training all over again, but this sergeant said, "Well, we're going to give you another chance."

So he called and told me he was going to take the test again on such and such a day. He had to cover this field running with full pack and rifle and bayonnet in so many minutes.

The day of the test came and the sergeant drove his jeep to the other end of the field and went to sleep. J. said, "I knew I was never going to make it and I was praying and asking the Hierarchy to help me and suddenly the man in the jeep woke up." When J. came up the sergeant went over to him and said, "I told the corporal to pass you because I knew you were going to fail again." He said, "I was sound asleep and somebody shook me by the shoulder and said, 'Get over there and get that boy through this test.' " He said, "I did it before I realized what I had done, but somebody spoke to me."

So J. told him what had happened, and thanked him for it and showed him his bead and said, "This was undoubtedly my Guru because I asked him to help me." The sergeant said, "Well, I don't want any of that stuff around here." J. said, "Well, I'll tell you this, someday when you are in trouble you will be helped because of the very fact that you helped the Hierarchy."

46. One of my disciples asked me tonight, "How can people reestablish the concept of Hierarchy, because that link seems to have been lost?"

A simple example of how that contact is made happened the other day. One of my students was coming to class and ran out of gas. Some Barnum and Baily Circus people came up and asked if they could help. She said, "Yes, I'd appreciate it very much." They got gas for her and were just wonderful. They said, "Where are you going?" She said, "I'm going to an Agni Yoga class." And they said, "How interesting. We wish we could go along with you." She said, "I wish you could too." "But," they said, "we have work to do; however, we'll go along in thought."

As she finished telling me the story, she said, "Wasn't that kind of them?" I said, "It was also kind of you to run out of gas. That was no accident. The fact that they helped you, they have been of service to the Hierarchy."

There is the story of an Englishman who found a co-worker of the Hierarchy lying unconscious on a mountain pass in the Himalayas. He had fallen and broken his hip. The Englishman carried him eight or nine miles to where he could get help and from that time on he and his family were under the protection of the Hierarchy because he had been of service.

On the other hand, when you represent the Hierarchy, don't be upset if people slander you or treat you badly, and don't look for revenge. They have caused the thing to happen and the Hierarchy will take care of that too. This is what Christ meant when he said, "Vengeance is mine, saith the Lord."

47. When you have developed every potential within you and have become perfected, then you are a Mahatma. Whatever talent you have, take that and develop it into two others. You should do three things extremely well as careers.

Count St. Germain could dictate seven letters in seven different languages on seven different subjects to seven different secretaries all at the same time as quickly as they could take them without losing the thread of what he was saying. It takes mastership over your mind, your thinking and your body. That's what Mahatmaship is.

This is why meditation is a very wonderful thing. If you can sit down for twenty minutes without moving a muscle, you are controlling your body. Every time you make an unnecessary movement you are wasting precious psychic energy. This is why the Indians will sit and not move. Our American Indians do the same thing or they will stand absolutely still and not move. They have learned to control the body.

The next step then is to learn to control the mind and not let it jump around like a monkey in a tree from branch to branch.

48. When you are writing something, dedicate it to Hierarchy and They will overshadow it. For instance, the movie, *The Day The Earth Stood Still,* is a very good example of how this is done.

I met the re-writer. The original writer was Bates, but the re-writer and I had lunch one day in Hollywood. We had a wonderful talk. He told me, "Originally, the story was about a robot who came to Earth from another planet and whose servant was a man. I changed it all around and made the man the master of the robot."

He wrote a speech in which the man, while talking to the Earth scientists, said, "We regret you cannot live in peace. You are behaving like children but that is your problem, and you must work it out." In other words that is your karma. "As long as you use your toy boats and planes and guns to kill each other, we cannot interfere but when you begin to endanger the other planets, we will have to destroy this one in order to preserve the planetary system."

This is one of Master Morya's speeches made about twenty-eight years ago, written down word for word, comma for comma. I said, "Where did you get this idea?" He said, "I don't know. It just came over me and it wrote itself." I told him a little about the Teaching and he said, "I can't tell you what it means to me to know that there exists a Brotherhood all over the world with no prejudice and no hatred—only love. It's a beautiful thing." He almost cried at the luncheon table, he was so overcome.

49. This Earth is a classroom, and if the people don't learn their lessons and graduate They'll "burn the school house down." We can't lag behind because some students are bad or stupid, while others are brilliant; it's not fair. The time has come. The Maitreya is here and ready or not the whole thing has to move. That is why there are so many difficulties and catastrophies and all this hate. These people will destroy one another.

But, if you are a person who brings harmony and peace and beauty into the lives of others, or makes this a better world through inventions, or helps the suffering of people, you are not going to be destroyed. Why would you be destroyed if you are a valuable worker for the Hierarchy? There are too few such workers who are willing to do this. For instance, many dedicated doctors and nurses are functioning unknowingly under the Hierarchy.

This is why we ask in our prayer for the blessing of all people who work consciously or unconsciously because many do work unconsciously. There is a gynecologist who takes special cases of women who have been told they need a hysterectomy. He will do anything rather than operate and he has saved countless women from this terrible surgery. People come to him from all over the world. His name is given to them by Master Morya for that particular purpose and reason. The doctor doesn't know who Master M. is or have any idea of the Hierarchy but the Hierarchy knows all about him and the word is passed from mouth to mouth. This is how it operates. You don't necessarily have to know. If you do, you can do that much more, although sometimes an instrument of Hierarchy is better off not knowing because the ego can become so involved they lose it.

The idea of healing is love. In the *Brown Brother* there is this beautiful statement, "The true essence of healing is the true essence of love and the true essence of love is the true essence of initiation." As Christ said, "Love one another." This is the key. Man has separated himself from God by saying this group or that group is no good, only our group is good. God has not separated Himself from them; they have separated themselves from Him.

50. The Hierarchy tests you in many ways and many times it's done in dreams. I can tell you about one of my tests. M. appeared and he had a little sack. He reached down into the sack and said, "Now, this is a solid gold object. It really belongs to a man named Miller but he doesn't know it. It's to go to him but if you take it he won't know the difference." I said, "No!" He said, "But it's very valuable," and I

said, "I don't care if it's valuable or not, I don't want it." He kept on insisting until finally I said, "No, I do not want it! Now please go away with it! I won't have it!" I had to get very tough about it.

About dreams—it's always significant when you dream about your Guru.

While we are on the subject of testing I must tell you this story. One evening I was dining with these very good friends of mine in New York. He was a connoisseur of wines and food and had this great wine cellar. He said, "R. will you have some wine?" and I said, "No, thank you, I can't drink alcohol. I get violently ill, but thank you very much." He said, "But these are very rare, very fine wines." I said, "Yes, thank you, but I can't drink any alcohol." So he kept insisting and insisting and I said, "Look, if you want to make me ill and if that will make you happy then I will drink it, but I don't want it and I think I've explained why." So he layed off.

Later his wife was telling me they had had another guest from England who was in the Arcane School and he went through this routine with her and said, "Oh, come on have some wine," and the woman said, no, she didn't drink, and he kept insisting and so she said, "Oh all right, I'll take a little," and just as she lifted the glass to her lips he said, "A fine metaphysician you are, drinking wine." It was really a vicious attack on her but it was also a test.

Actually everything is a test. One time I was between decorating jobs and had about three dollars in the bank. My rent and everything was paid but I was really down very low.

Earlier I was called in on a healing in which both the man and his wife were psychiatrists. She had been very ill for a long time and I had been treating her for about two months when they called me and said she was completely well. They knew the payment was to help twenty or thirty people and they said they would take twenty people a year who were in poor circumstances and give them a whole psychiatric treatment. So this was even more than I had expected, but then he wrote a check and left the amount blank and said I could fill it in up to ten thousand dollars.

I said, "This is not the way it works. We are not allowed to accept money for a healing." He said, "I know, but you could use it to help other people," and I said, "No, I'm sorry, but that is the rule." And when he wouldn't take it back, I tore up the check.

I went home and there was a telephone call for me and I got this big decorating job. This was also a test. I could have rationalized this thing, because that's very easy to do, but this is where you have to be very rigid. It's either yes or no. It's really walking the razor's edge. There is no deviation from right or wrong. It's all the way or nothing.

Many times in the Teaching people complain that I'm too strict. I say, "No, I'm not strict. The Hierarchy is strict, and if you're going to work with the Hierarchy, it's all or nothing."

Or, someone may call and ask for help and you're very, very busy. It's easy to say, "I'm too busy today, I'll do it tomorrow," but the fact that they called you at that moment is reason enough to set aside what you were doing and go and help. That's also a test. Or if you see an accident happen before you, that means God has put you there as His servant and it's your duty to help.

Mahatmas

51. What the Mahatmas do on occasion is leave their physical bodies in Shambhala and go astrally to either Jupiter or Venus or the higher planets and work there on wisdom and knowledge and bring it back with them. It's like a sacred retreat. And while they are away, another brother in Shambhala takes care of their body.

While we are on the subject of Mahatmas, there is a beautiful story that was told to me by Natalie Kalmus, of the color film people. She was brought to my studio in New York and we talked. She said, "Many years ago up on the farm in New Hampshire we had very severe winters. My sister, who was sixteen at the time, was very delicate and couldn't walk. She had been paralyzed since she was twelve. There was no television to entertain us in those days so my father was a great reader, and on winter evenings when we were snowed-in we would all read a different book about the same period in history. For instance, one of us would read about Catherine the Great of Russia, another about King Frederick of Prussia and another would read Voltaire and about the King of France and the King of England, all in the same period, and then we would compare notes and discuss this."

She said, "My father always said no one was to be turned away from his door for want of food and if they wanted shelter they could stay in the barn. So," she said, "consequently we always had tramps." She said, "This was a particularly wild winter night and the snow was drifting and we had just gone into the living room and started our usual game of putting all of these books together. The cook came in and said there was a man at the door who wanted food and since she had just cleaned everything up and was tired, what did we want her to do with him?'' "My father said, 'I'll take care of him. You go do what you want.' So my father went out into the kitchen and this man was a very attractive individual, well dressed but shabby, and he asked for food and shelter. So,'' she said, ''my father fixed him a dinner and while he ate my father was reading this book. He thought he wouldn't leave him alone but would keep an eye on him. The man continued to eat and then he said, 'That's a very interesting book but the facts are not all correct.' 'It happens to be about the court of France,' and the man said, 'Yes, I know. On such and such page there is a passage'— and he quoted it—'that's totally incorrect. It was inserted by someone who just made it up, and in the fourth chapter, third paragraph there is a passage and that is erroneous. That didn't happen at all and this is what took place...' My father said, 'Are you a writer?' and the man said, 'No, I write a great deal, but I don't profess to be a writer.' 'But,' my father said, 'you question this.' The man said, 'Let's say I'm a historian and I collect facts and this book is in error.' 'Now,' he said, 'that book over there about Catherine the Great of Russia is extremely correct, except for two points in it that are in error.' My father asked him, 'What are they?' The man said, 'It's about the two visitors who came to the court. In the book they mention these two men were adventurers, but they were not, they were Mahatmas.' '' Of course, as we all know, Count St. Germain and Cagliostro went to her court in Russia.

And she told me, "My father knew nothing of this or about the Hierarchy, and the conversation went on and one and when the man had finished my father asked him, 'Would you come in and meet my family?' So he came in and the man was charming and entertaining and he spoke beautiful English with no colloquial accent. He held them spellbound and when it came time to go to bed my father said, 'Would you like to take our guest room?' The man said, 'How do you know I wouldn't murder you all in the middle of the night?' My father said, 'I trust you,' and the man said, 'Thank you, I'd be delighted to stay.'

"Now, up to this point the man had never even looked at my sister who was sitting in the wheel chair, but as he was going upstairs and saying goodnight he put his hand on her shoulder and said, 'Tomorrow morning you will walk again.' The family thought this was the collapse of a beautiful evening, a very cruel thing to do to this youngster who hadn't walked in four years.'' And she said, ''We all went to bed with heavy hearts.

"The next morning we were waiting for our guest to come down and finally my father went up and knocked on the door. When there was no answer, he went in and the bed had not been slept in. All the doors and windows were locked from the inside. There were no tracks in the snow where he had left, and there was no stranger. And, my sister got up and walked.

"Well, my father was very excited. He got out the sleigh and drove around the countryside in a radius of about eight miles inquiring about this stranger, and finally he found one farmhouse where the woman said, 'Oh yes, a stranger came about two o'clock in the morning and asked for food. My baby was dying of pneumonia and I had called and begged the doctor to come, but he wouldn't come because the snow was so bad.' So the stranger said, 'Let me hold the baby while you're fixing some food.' And she said, 'The baby went to sleep in his arms and was soon breathing normally. He ate his food and said thank you and disappeared.' ''

This was a Mahatma, and these things often happen.

52. One of the most amazing and exciting stories I've ever heard was a demonstration by Count and Countess Cagliostro and Count St. Germain, in which they invited twenty-two living people to a chateau outside of Paris and they asked each one to name any dead and brilliant person they would like to have as their dinner partner. Of course the dead didn't eat.

The twenty-two guests came down to dinner, and at each place these various people from the past were sitting. Catherine the Great and mad Ludwig and so forth were sitting there and they talked back and forth with the living. And then these twenty-two living people said it was a trick.

It was one of the most spectacular things that Mahatmas ever did. It was the astral body of these people that came. The astral body is just like the physical, and They materialized the astral to prove that death does not exist. All of this is recorded and definitely happened.

This was before the French Revolution. Ben Franklin was there and he was very impressed, but then he was already a Mahatma. You see, Franklin, Adams, George Washington, Jefferson, all of these men were of the White Brotherhood. All of the men who signed the Declaration of Independence were either Adepts or Mahatmas—great men. This is when our country was very exciting. Now, when you study the history of America and its forefathers and then compare that with today, what have you got?—nothing!

53. There was a legend that George Washington was the Mahatma who would be the father of our country. Look at the way they fought the British and French troops and the Germans, who were all beautifully equipped with guns and money, and we had nothing. Washington's men wore bags on their feet because they had no shoes. They had no guns so they used pitch forks. They were fighting for

great freedoms, freedom of speech and freedom of religion, in which people were going to be allowed to worship God in any form they wanted without persecution. This was the New World. This is why we won and this is why we had a Mahatma leading us.

Wherever there is a need a Mahatma is sent to help. There was a story written up in the *New York Times* some years ago about a closed meeting that was being held at the United Nations late one night. It was around midnight and all the doors were locked to the spectators gallery and they were having a real fight among themselves and couldn't reach an agreement when suddenly this tall man in Oriental robes and turban stood up in the balcony and said, "Gentlemen, gentlemen, the situation is this..." and "the solution is this...," and in about fifteen words he presented the problem and its solution. They applauded and he bowed, and with that he disappeared right before their eyes. The doors were all locked and there were no guards, and no one came and no one left. This is the way They operate.

54. One day this lady called me and said, "R., I have this growth the size of a grapefruit and I can't walk, and the doctors tell me it's a tumor but they don't know if its benign or what it is and I've got to do something fast. The doctors have suggested an immediate operation." I said, "Call your doctor and ask if you can have just ten days." So she did, and he said, "Yes, ten days won't make much difference one way or the other." So we began treatment, and she went back in ten days and it was the size of an orange. In another week it was the size of a plum, then it became the size of a cherry and then the size of a pea and then it was dissolved.

So you know this was a pretty terrific individual. She did fashion work in New York and was a very beautiful, sophisticated woman, a very wonderful person.

She was telling me this story later. She said, "I was doing a fashion show in New Haven, Connecticut and it went very well. I always dedicated everything to the Hierarchy. After the show a lot of people wanted to take me to a party at the home of one of their friends. I said, 'I don't drink, but I'll have a glass of gingerale with you.' I was so tired I felt like going to the hotel and to bed, but I thought I'll go and sit quietly and rest. There were about twenty-five people there and we got to talking about philosophy and I just sat back and said, 'Dear God, I'm out of this. I'm so tired and I don't want to get involved with all these strangers anyway.' Then this boy got up and said, 'I feel I create my own life. There is no God, no destiny, nothing. You create everything yourself.'

I found myself saying, 'Either you are a very wise man or a very stupid one,' and for the next two hours the words just came out of me and I talked about the Hierarchy and God and I just sat there amazed at the things that were coming out of me, things I didn't even know.'' This boy came to New York, they had lunch together; he bought all the books of the Teaching and has been studying Agni Yoga ever since.

This is what happens many times; one of the Hierarchy will take over and use you and you are the mouth and they are the sound that comes out, especially if you are challenged by a group of people. This was no accident. He was put there and she was put there for that purpose. Nothing is by accident, but all is by a beautiful design.

55. Mahatmas can only work with certain levels of people. For instance, if They came into the presence of a very low consciousness with Their consciousness being so much higher, it would kill that person. They don't want to do that. They want live workers. What They must do, then, is raise the consciousness of that individual and lower Theirs, but They are not going to approach a third root race person to do this. They are going to approach a fifth or six race person because these are the people who have been brought in to speed up the evolution of the planet.

The Mahatmas will never work through organized groups where they charge a fee or where any money is involved, never! Or if someone advertises that he is working through a certain Mahatma, this is not true. A Mahatma will never do this, nor will they ever work through a spiritualist or medium, never! If a spiritualist tells you they are going to manifest a Mahatma, don't believe them, they can't do it.

No Mahatma will ever sign a book, so if you find a book signed by a Mahatma, question it immediately. There is a third edition of *The Secret Doctrine* in which you will find six thousand errors. This is not put out by the Theosophy group but by a private printing press, for profit. Be warned and be careful. You have volume one and volume two of *The Secret Doctrine* and volume one and two of *Isis Unveiled*. In one of the volumes of *The Secret Doctrine* it mentions that Madame Blavatsky started a third book and this is true but she died before it was finished. Someone else took the manuscripts and manufactured the rest. All you have to do is check with the Theosophists and ask if this is a spurious book and they will tell you, yes.

In the writing of *The Mahatma Letters,* They worked directly. For instance, letters would appear on the pillow. The Mahatmas will work directly with you as well. Sometimes they will work through your Guru if there is a need.

If they are suspected of being a Mahatma they will disappear and reappear in another place.

56. Suppose you were a Mahatma and you were reborn in this body into an ordinary family with the full knowledge of who you were. How could you take it? You couldn't possibly. So what They have to do is block out certain things and dim certain memories until you are able to cope with them and put it all into its proper place. Then it's given to you, but until that particular time you would go mad with the responsibility of knowing who and what you were. As a child, for instance, you wouldn't fit in anywhere.

This happened to HPB. They withdrew part of this knowledge. It was also true of JFK, because as you know, he was George Washington. It was the prophesy that he would return, but not with his complete memory. Part of that memory was retained; that part of his consciousness that was kept back was stored in Shambhala. It's part of the spirit, not the soul. Certain personality traits come in with you. For instance, his ability to read the press from all over the world. This is a very unusual thing. Both John and his wife and Robert were very unique people in every sense of the word. So, they have all come in with these special qualities and other qualities have been kept back until they reach a certain level and then it can be given to them.

This is only true of fifth and sixth root race people. As a further example, take Frank Lloyd Wright, and Edison and Tesla and Marconi. All of these men, these geniuses, were misunderstood, and Einstein too until he proved his theory. They were laughed at and ridiculed because they were fifth and sixth root race peple living among threes and fours. How many people can you talk to and converse with on an esoteric level outside of the Teaching? Only a handful.

57. When the Mahatmas appear they densify by lowering their vibratory rate and lift your vibrations up so there is a balance. Otherwise, they would kill you. You will never see a Mahatma until you are ready. They will appear when you least expect it and it will be so ordinary that two or three days will elapse before you realize this was an unusual event and then you will get a reaction.

There is a very interesting story of how we got the pictures of the Mahatmas for the shrine. They came to me through old Dr. Ramas who, at 98, was still in practice with Dr. Ryan, who was 108. Their hours were 9 to 6 and they took only cancer, leukemia, multiple sclerosis and diseases like that.

As a young man Dr. Ramas was on his way to Vienna to study medicine when he met an old sea captain who showed him some beautiful paintings of the Mahatmas on silk and opened up this whole esoteric thing to him, and Dr. Ramas became very interested in Theosophy and the Masters. When the captain died, he left these paintings to Dr. Ramas who in turn loaned them to us.

Then there was the question of whether we should have these pictures on the shrine for people to see. Finally the Mahatmas said, "Yes, We will grant this because the vibrations from these pictures are so beneficial that people should be exposed to them."

When Dr. Ramas died, the pictures went to one of his relatives, so we had to give them up, but we asked permission to photograph them and these are the reproductions we have now.

These two doctors were completely devoted to service. Dr. Ramas knew when a patient was going to die, and he would go to the bedside and pray them through Devachan. Dr. Ryan had studied medicine in Tibet and spent many years practicing in Siberia. While there he discovered how to make a yogurt that would rejuvenate the tissues. This is actually what preserved his vitality and life for so many years.

Mrs. Ramas, who was much younger than her husband, told me her story. She said, "I never approved of this thing my husband was into, doing all these meditations, and although I had great respect and love for him, I thought this is his plaything. One night we were in a hotel room in Rome and my husband had to go out for something. I was pregnant with our first child and felt swollen and uncomfortable and I was feeling sorry for myself and I began to cry. Suddenly," she said, "I felt someone in the room and I turned and there was M. and He said, 'Stop that this instant.' " She said, "Believe me, I did." He appeared to her and that's all he said, and from then on she was devoted to the Teaching.

So when we talk about the Mahatmas, don't think they are away off somewhere looking down at us wondering if we're going to make it. They are in our daily lives. They are in our cities, in our towns, and I quote the Teaching, "We use plane tickets, train tickets, boat tickets. We walk about in the cities, in the villages, everywhere, at all times." They are extremely sympathetic and interested in everyone who is aware of something beyond themselves, and you never know when a Mahatma will appear. The moment you become interested in any form of esoteric work or Teaching or in changing your consciousness, a battery of lights is focused on you and from that moment on They (the Mahatmas) are watching your thoughts, your mind, your actions and reactions and They are trying to help you. They say, "We are your shield."

58. Various fragrances have specific associations. For instance, fresh violets are always associated with Father Pio, and when Morya is near you will always smell roses, even if there are no roses in the room, or sandalwood incense. One night we were driving to Trenton,

New Jersey, and talking about these things and the whole car was filled with the heaviest aroma of sandalwood. Of course, no one was burning incense and even though it was a very cold night we had to open the windows because it was so overpowering.

As I've said before, when you go to the museum you're going to the house of the muses. Some time ago I took a woman from India to the museum and we were standing in front of a statue of Buddha from Nepal, and she said, "Mr. H., can you smell that scent?" and I said, "Yes," and she said, "That is the odor of a particular kind of primrose that only grows in the northern part of India where I was born and raised. Later I moved to Calcutta and I have never smelled that fragrance since then until we stood in front of this statue." The odor was pouring in like fresh flowers.

It is possible that the frangrance of sandalwood can also be attributed to K.H. because M. and K.H. work very closely together. They have houses back to back with a connecting garden and a bridge over a stream. They work together in the old form of Buddhism. I have a very ancient plate some four or five hundred years old, and on it there is a drawing with two gardens and a bridge and this man is under a tree and up in the corner is the form of two people. This pictures the Subtle World, meaning "as above, so below."

59. If a Dhyan Chohan has finished the work He came here to do and wants to go back to His original planet and rest there for a while, in so doing that experience would be wiped from His memory, although it would remain in the seed of the spirit. The consciousness would be there but the memory would be dimmed.

Just like a Mahatma who returns here to do work on the Earth. If He came in with full memory of His Mahatmaship, who would He be able to talk to or have anything to do with? Imagine being born into a family and trying to explain the various laws of Hierarchy to them. You couldn't, and they'd think you were absolutely insane, and you'd have no communication with anyone. So the memory of having been a Mahatma is wiped away like an eraser across a blackboard; not completely, but blurred.

A Dhyan Chohan has earned the right to go back to his planet and rest after serving 550 million years. He may be tired and want to go back. Not everyone has the chance to become a Dhyan Chohan, but then not everyone will do anything about anything. It's like the Teaching; I've been in this work since I was sixteen and we only have a handful of people here and there. We have groups all over but we only have small numbers in each group.

60. Many times people will ask me, "Why do you call the Mahatmas by initials, like M or KH or HPB?" When you speak the

name of an individual you call them in psychically. There's a connection somewhat like a radio wave. By using Their initials you don't pull in Their ray and this is showing consideration for Them. You should not pull Them in unless They are needed, as They are very busy people. Sometimes in meetings we deliberately use the name of the Masters to bring in that ray for the benefit of the people there.

Some of the Mahatmas' names are not given out because they would be misused, like misusing a mantram. It's like hearing about a mantram and saying I'll use it anyway even though I don't need it. It's opening Pandora's box; you can't close it again.

Mantrams and things like that are very sacred and very powerful. One must have a healthy respect for them. "Aum" is a very good mantram. It's constructive and one you can always use. It sets up a whole vibratory rate but will never be harmful. There is a legend that if you utter the word Aum in the Ajanta Caves in India, you will hear the voice of Buddha. Also for singers, Aum is a perfect placement for the tone. It cannot be placed in the throat. The mantram "Aum Tat Sat Aum" loosely translated means "The Dew Is On The Lotus." We are like the dew drop and the lotus represents God.

"Shanti" is the Sanskrit word for Peace.

"Vishnu Shakti" is also often used. "Shakti" is the word for "center" or "movement," and Vishnu was the first Avatar. He reincarnated as Rama, as Krishna, as Shiva, as Moses, and all the way down until the thirteenth incarnation He became Buddha. This is why Vishnu is a very powerful name to use. When we say "Vishnu Shakti" we are bringing in all thirteen Avatars and the fourteenth will be the Lord Maitreya.

61. As the Teachings say, and I quote from *The Mahatma Letters,* "No married man or woman can be a Mahatma," unless it is arranged by their Guru that they have a special union for the purpose of having children after which they are husband and wife in name only.

There are very special circumstances—like the Roerichs and their two sons. They were together for that particular purpose to bring in these two children. George died in Russia. There were seventy-five paintings that had been lost for thirty or forty years and I discovered them out on the West Coast. They were of all the old castles and holy places of Russia that Roerich had done as a young man in 1904. Originally, they were going to be put into a special museum by Czar Nicholas, so when they were found George was asked to bring them back to Russia. He did, they had lunch, and he died right after lunch. Svetoslav lives in India. He is the artist and also a Guru.

62. The ring of the Mahatmas that they speak about is made of

silver and set with turquoise. It is no longer made of gold. This is the ring of Gessar Khan's castle. The Mahatmas wear it or give it as a present.

There is another jewel that many of you have probably read about. It is the Agni pearl. If you ask any jeweler who knows pearls for an Agni pearl, he will tell you they are almost impossible to obtain. There are only a limited number of them in the world. They are a fresh water pearl and look like black patent leather.

The girl who did the illustrations for my little book, *White Jade,* received one. It was given to her. It is always given. They are worth a great sum of money, but this one was given to her in Hong Kong by a Chinese man who told her, "This is a present and you must never sell it or give it away." With that ring she got into Tibet; she got into the holy places of Turkey and India and throughout the East. As soon as these holy men saw she was wearing it the doors were open to her, because they knew she had earned it. That's the only way you can get it.

63. King Alexander was working directly with the Mahatmas, and all the Greek philosophers except Socrates went to Egypt to the mystery schools and were initiated by Isis in Egypt, and then they all went to Tibet.

64. The Venetian Master was the great painter Veronese.

65. Count and Countess Cagliostro and Count St. Germain were Mahatmas. They appeared in every court in Europe and played tremendously great dramatic roles in the history of France, Russia, Prussia, England and Holland.

They worked with Catherine the Great of Russia to open clinics for the poor. They knew medicines. They knew alchemy. They built many hospitals, and spent vast sums of money to help the poor.

They guided the destinies of all these nations and warned them of impending dangers. All of the revolutions could have been avoided. It wasn't meant that they should be democracies but that they should be kingdoms. The kings and queens and emperors and empresses were born for the karma of that country, to rule wisely and well, and if they would rule in this manner they could bring their country to greatness.

For instance, the Czar was always called "the little father of all the Russias" because he had divine right, and when the people came to him and asked him to give up this divine right he wouldn't do it. Instead of that, when he went off to the front to fight in the war, he gave that divine right to Alexandra who was a German and the people hated her. This is what caused the revolution.

Queen Victoria was also given advice by the Mahatmas. Both M.

and K.H. visited her in the trappings of an Indian Prince at the time of her Golden Jubilee and begged her not to do certain things or she would lose her colonies and England would fall on hard times. But instead of doing the right thing, she allowed England to become politically involved with China, and they brought opium into that country and this brought on a whole karmic disaster. Look at England today. We are in the process of seeing the entire Empire crumble.

Spain crumbled with the Inquisition. One of their leaders had only one eye, and with that eye he could see the devil in people, and if you had a big estate he saw the devil very quickly and the Church took it over and that was that. So you see when you violate cosmic law you pay for it, and today Spain is still the beggar in the dust. Once it was the greatest nation on Earth.

One of the best books written about Count St. Germain is by Cooper Oakley. Unfortunately it's out of print. In this book they tell about the Yusupov Family. It was Alexis Yusupov who killed Rasputin. St. Germain was a great friend of the family. I knew the family later on and one day I said, "It must have been wonderful to know St. Germain," and he said, "Not interested."

I asked the Queen of Holland if she knew Count St. Germain. I asked her this direct question because I know He is in her court. This I know, so I said, "Do you know a man named Count St. Germain?" and she just looked at me and smiled. I said, "Do you know him?" and she said, "Lovely weather, isn't it?" I couldn't get anything out of her at all but she looked very knowingly and had a twinkle in her eye. One of my disciples in Rome was dying to get on a plane and go to Holland to see if we could find him, but I said, "No, this is very wrong. Unless you have been sent for, you shouldn't do it."

You see, there have been healers in that court for some time. The mother of Queen Wilhemena was an initiate and both Queen Frederika of Greece and her husband were disciples of Roerich. Old King Leopold was also a disciple of Roerich and these people knew what they were doing.

The anointing of kings and queens, emperors and empresses is based on the idea of opening their clairvoyance so they can rule their countries with all their senses, including their sixth sense.

The stone under the throne chair of the king or queen is a very sacred stone. It's a magnet, a lodestone, but the actual mystery of it has been lost, and it remains only a stone.

Many a king wanders the Earth in beggar's rags for things done and left undone. Being a king is a very tough assignment because they are in charge of the karma of that whole country. That's why they say heavy is the head that wears the crown. It's a tremendous responsibility. The crown is basically the crown of achievement of the spirit.

The jewels in the crown are there for the purpose of warding off the negative influences of the planets or for protection when the country is going through a bad period of time. It's not that the diamonds or emeralds or rubies are valuable but it means each jewel gives off an emanation which is related to a specific planet and the jewels are worn to offset these planetary influences.

Even today those of you who are initiates wear a jewel to protect you. That's your teraphim. Topaz actually throws off an energy and is very beneficial for the health of old people or people who are weak and don't have much energy. Rubies have a certain use and so on, and this creates a balance. All of these legends are based on truths and when you know and work with them you benefit.

66. At the time of the crucifixion of Christ his last words were, "My God, why hast thou forsaken me?" In that instant he attained Mahatmaship, because when you are on the edge of the abyss help comes and only then. Put yourself in his position and you too would cry out. It was his humaness that caused him to cry out, but in that moment something happened and he became a Mahatma. He had everything else, but there was that little personal fear of life and death and as soon as it came out in the open he finished that part of his karma and could go on.

Mahatma Letters

67. The book *The Mahatma Letters* was compiled from letters that were written by the Mahatmas M. and K.H. to A.P. Sinnett in the late 1800's in answer to questions from Sinnett. The original hand-written manuscripts can be found in The British Museum in London. (In the English Manuscript section.)

I have often been asked how we can go about writing a letter to the Mahatmas. What you do is write your letter and put whatever you want into it and then you burn it and let the ashes go out the window. It goes out into space and will reassemble itself for the Mahatmas.

In *The Mahatma Letters* They tell you that many times you will receive your answer in an envelope on your pillow. It is received in the same way it is sent. All the Mahatma letters were received in that way and they came in the middle of winter to England accompanied by a beautiful red rose. They don't guarantee you will always get an answer right away, but when the answer comes it will be in this manner.

You can also write down a question, any question that is of a serious nature affecting yourself and the Teaching, and address it to your Guru. The answer will come psychically and when you get it, check it with your Guru to see if it is right. This establishes that rapport and link between you and the more you do it the stronger that link becomes.

Kumaras

68. There is a whole Hierarchy of Kumaras. Each of us come under a separate Kumara, and you will work under the rays of that Kumara. All those who are from Venus would come under one Kumara. All those from another planet come under another Kumara. It's a Hierarchy of Kumaras working together like the Hierarchy of Mahatmas.

Number one, we are operating with our Guru, then with our Mahatma, then with the Dhyan Choan, then with the Kumaras, and then with the Lords of Karma. It's a complete thing like a network of wires on a switchboard. It would be very good to link with each of these spirits.

But you see, the Guru cannot instruct people to do these things. We can give hints and then the individual has to do a little more. If you are told to do something it will lose its effect, but if you can do it on your own, then you will get results. Always do more than you are asked to do. Do a little extra if you can see something else to be done.The fact that you can get an idea and act on it means you are moving in the right direction.

An artist who strives for a new art form will be helped by their Kumara because they are bringing beauty and culture into the world. Or, suddenly the Lords of Karma will give all the accumulations of someone who has dropped the ball to another individual who is striving. If you link with Them and strive to pick up the indications, They will do great and wonderful things for you.

69. Each Kumara is dedicated to a particular planet for a

manvantara—which is 550 million years—and is responsible for everyone on it. When there is a new planet, another Kumara takes the responsibility of that planet upon himself for the whole length of time. A Kumara comes from another planetary system. The Maitreya, the Manu and the Kumara are all from other planetary systems.

Kumaras are similar to but higher than a Planetary Spirit because They take on a new planet, whereas the Planetary Spirit takes on a planet already conceived. Lucifer was a Kumara who went wrong. He could also be called an archangel. The fall of Lucifer held back the evolution of Earth at least ten thousand years.

A Manu is in charge of a solar system. Our Manu is one of the great souls who is in charge of our solar system. He is head of it.

70. The Lord Maitreya is more than one consciousness. He is part of the consciousness of Christ, part of the consciousness of Buddha, of Rama, of Vishnu, of Moses, of all the great holy men that go back into time, of all the religions, of all the great Teachers. He is the Truth of each one of them. He is the essence of their souls. And He is coming from another planetary system than ours.

The Lord Maitreya is the new Kumara of the Earth. He is actually higher than a Planetary Spirit, and because of this we can experience a direct teaching of cosmic laws.

This Teaching will never be for all people. I quote, "We send you the people and none comes by error and if it appears they come by error, it is meant they are to be exposed to it for the next life." We are the sowers. We sow the seeds on rocks, on fertile ground, on barren ground, but never worry where the seed falls for the wind will carry it to a place where it will grow and it will become fertile and bloom. We are but the gardeners. You go and look at the garden once in a while and if it needs attention you give it, but you have done your duty when you sow.

Before Lord Maitreya, Lucifer was the Kumara and look how he mucked it up. We have not been without a Kumara, we have been with a negative one, one who went mad over power. In 1936 his power came to an end, but there are still enough dark ones to keep things muddled and going. Many of us were put here to unbalance what he has been doing. If a negative condition exists because of Lucifer, the Mahatmas will put someone here to counteract this influence, but they cannot change him as that would be interfering with karma.

Roerich, N.K.

71. The Pact and Banner of Peace was conceived by Nicholas Roerich. The symbol for it is a large red circle, the color of roses, on a white background; inside the circle are three red dots in the form of a triangle with the first dot on top. The red circle means immortality, life everlasting. The three dots mean Guru, Guide and Master; it also means Father, Son and Holy Ghost; or Science, Art and Religion. These are all one. Now, Roerich designed this to be a flag which would fly over all the art museums, schools, colleges, hospitals, public libraries and historical places; over all the treasures of the world in every country. He began this project in 1936 and had succeeded in persuading many of the nations of the world to sign a pact agreeing, in case of war, not to bomb any building flying this flag, because these were treasures belonging to the world. He was to have won the Nobel Prize for peace, but in 1939 Hitler declared war and the whole idea was abandoned.

This is a very ancient symbol found in Tibet; on the coat of arms of the Popes in Rome; on Messerling's Christ in Antwerp, right over the heart; in Spain; on Japanese armor; in the Temple of Heaven in Peking, on the dome and on the floor, signifying as above so below; it was seen on the Gobi desert; on the swords of Gessar Khan; in Africa; in South America; in Germany; in Sweden and Finland. It's purely an international symbol, very ancient, as old as the Earth, and I quote Roerich, "It belongs to no sect, or group or person but to the universe." That is why He chose this symbol to fly over the treasures of the world. They belong to the cultured people of the world and should never be destroyed.

Today the underground symbol of peace is the inverted Y within a circle, but these three dots within a circle are being used as the above ground symbol of peace.

72. Morya designed the Master's Institute (in New York City) and it was built during the Depression. It was to go up eleven stories and have a stupa on top. Stupas are found in Tibet. They are round and on the top is a cap that is filled with a measured amount of water. At the end of the year they open this and if there is more water, this is a bad omen and means war. If there is less water, this is a good omen.

But instead of the stupa, the architect ran the building up another twenty-seven stories and put a restaurant on top.

It was designed as a place where creative people in all fields of art could come and live and work. It was a great success for several years until Roerich went to the Gobi desert to get two ship loads of grass seed to plant in the dust bowls of the Midwest. It was the kind of grass that would grow on top of sand and prevent the top soil from shifting. The ships arrived, but (a high government official) had the seeds dumped into the harbor.

No, Roerich was not interfering with the karma of the people in the dust bowl, even though out of their greed they turned the prairie into wheat fields and then when the price of wheat went down abandoned the land; because when you see a disaster area or people in trouble, you go and help. If I am walking down the street and I see a child drowning, I'm not going to say, I won't help that child, it's his karma. I must go and help that child no matter who or what color he is because that's why I am there, to help.

73. The role that Judas played goes back to the whole idea of karma. The fact that he was given a chance over and over again to transcend his karma is a wonderful thing. For instance, my Guru knew that one of his disciples would betray him, yet he took him as a disciple because there was a chance that he would make it and if he did he would be very important to the Brotherhood. If you know there is betrayal in an individual, you can look at it and watch it, but you do not deny them the privilege of help in any way. As long as they are trying they must be given every opportunity, because the making of a member of the Brotherhood is more important than the possibility of betrayal. Judas will be given another chance to betray or not, because basically his essence is very wonderful or he wouldn't have been a disciple of Jesus.

What makes people betray? Power, money, position or some particular combination of these. Roerich was betrayed for eight million dollars, and people will say, "I wouldn't do that," but I tell them, "Don't say that, for how do you know until someone has offered you eight million dollars?" I hope to God I wouldn't do it, but I don't know myself that well. I don't think anyone does. You can't blame people for doing these things. This is their weakness and you don't know where your weakness is.

These traitors pay for their acts over and over again. Once I was at a political dinner at one of the hotels and this man came over and threw thirty dimes at the plate of the man who betrayed my Guru. It was the most shocking and ugly thing I've ever seen. He turned deathly white and got up and left.

If Judas had not betrayed Christ, we might never have had Christianity. He served a purpose. As Akbar said, "use your enemies for table legs." Sometimes people play ugly roles, and the Hierarchy will use that individual for a purpose. We should never judge because the Lords of Karma are watching and can superimpose these people to act as a catalyst.

As an illustration of this, at one time before I went to the coast (California) we had a very close knit group. It was a closed group, but one of the women became very difficult. I said, "Let's see what we are going to learn from this because there is a reason for everything." What it did was bring the rest of the group closer together than ever before and out of that group came this very wonderful idea of The Pantheon of Peace, a tremendous thing for the Brotherhood.

I went and thanked her for what she had done. She had been put there for that purpose. She was used and could have drawn merit for it. As Akbar said, "Who are my illustrious enemies today?" And he used them for his work.

Shambhala

74. Shambhala is a place. It exists in the mundane world and in the Fiery World. It is in Nepal beyond the mountain of Karikal. It is a complete city in which the Mahatmas dwell and people go there in spirit and some people like Master Roerich, my Guru, for instance, went there in the physical body. You cannot get in unless you are spiritually qualified. You must be summoned and if you try to make it on your own, you will be stopped.

In your dreams when you are ready to go to Shambhala this will happen: there will be a group of monks, seven or eight feet tall, and there will be a very large fire. From this fire one of the monks will take a knife and cut the sign of Vishnu in your arm and there is blood. This is Rigden Jeppo and this is your first initiation into Shambhala. You are not actually cut but in the dream you see and feel three lines down and two across and this is the sign of Vishnu.

The Lords of Shambhala are the Mahatmas. It is a very common thing for people who are disciples to be referred to as Princes and Princesses of Shambhala. This is the idea of possessing a nobility of spirit, and the wealth and great jewels given to the disciples are wisdom.

Nepal was opened to visitors about ten years ago for the first time in five thousand years. Previously, you went by invitation of the king who was a clairvoyant.

In the book *Lost Horizon,* by James Hilton, you have the whole story of Shambhala, but it's called Shangri-la. In it they mention the mountain of Karikal, and the old lama who was 108 years old—108 being a Tibetan mystical number—and how they prolonged life through love, and about the young Englishman, old in spirit from many lifetimes, who was to replace the old lama. It's all there.

You can go in the subtle body but only when you have developed to that point where you are accepted and invited.

One of my disciples in California wrote me this letter in which he told about this very wonderful dream. He said he was in a store buying this very mundane thing like a curtain rod for the bathroom and he told the clerk, "No, I want something more antique," and the floor manager said, "Well, if you want something like that you should go to Morya's castle." And he said, "Morya's castle? Do you know where that is?" And the man said, "Yes, it's up in the Hollywood hills." My disciple said, "I would love to go," and the next thing they were in the castle. The man said, "All right, I'll leave you now." And my disciple said it was like twilight and he was looking at all the things and he noticed that all the furniture was carved with the initial M on it, and there were beautiful things of art and suddenly all the lights came on and the whole castle lit up. Just before the lights came on, he opened a drawer and there was a painting of Akbar, the great Indian Emperor who later became Morya. He lit a match to look at this miniature painting and of course he knew who it was.

As you work and evolve and strive, you too will experience these things because they're not very far away.

75. The yellow peril has been mentioned all down through the ages. Always this has been the boogyman of the East, but actually it refers to the Oriental philosophy that is sweeping all over the world. The warriors are the holy men who are doing this work; warriors for truth, warriors for beauty, warriors for freedom from all despair and hatred and prejudice. This is the yellow peril that man is so frightened of. It means the release of man from the slavery of an unfulfilled spirit. This is the prophesy: that the banners of Shambhala will fly over all the world and this great and beautiful philosophy will open up the hearts of all people and the world will be completely changed.

Many of the present movements are the breaking down of the old forms; Shiva, Shiva, Shiva, the destroyer of the old, the antiquated, and the useless and the birth of that which is new and bright and shiny and tomorrow.

We are all warriors of Shambhala. It is our job to bring light and illumination to people. Wherever there is injustice we are expected to fight it for the benefit of all people. This is the Eastern occult form of God that is sweeping the country. There was a prophesy that the Eastern armies would come to the West. This army is made up of warriors who are flooding the land with all these ideas of karma and reincarnation and love for one another and respect for all religions and creeds, and they are battling to eliminate all this ugliness and greed.

The warriors of Shambhala are often spoken of as Princes and Princesses of spirit because you have to be dedicated to do this work of trying to build a better world. We are not to tear down the old and leave it but we must create a better one. Like the ancient Egyptians and Chaldeans and Mayans, who never tore down a temple but built another one over it. Strangely enough the Catholic Church has done the same thing. They have built over all the ancient Greek Temples such as the Temple of Venus and the Temple of Diana. They never tore down an altar—because it was a sacred thing—but built another one right over it and in this way they used all the emanations of these holy places. Wherever there is devotion and concentration there is tremendous power, and the early Church fathers knew this and used it.

Straight Knowledge

76. To get a "reading," Straight Knowledge is used. It works like a ticker tape right out in front of you so you can read it. When you have Straight Knowledge, you have access to the knowledge of the Mahatmas.

Straight Knowledge gives you the answer to any occult question that relates to our planet or planetary system, but the knowledge of infinity—no, we don't have that yet. You see, even our Mahatmas are confined to our solar system until They finish Their work and then They will operate in other solar systems. This is why man is going out into space.

Straight Knowledge is earned through many, many lifetimes.

Overshadowing

77. When the Mahatmas overshadow an Adept or you as an individual, it's as if you are the pencil and the Hierarchy is the lead. This is where your Straight Knowledge comes from. It's part of your development.

Any person who is leading an (Agni Yoga) group can be overshadowed if they so desire. It will never be inflicted by the Guru or the Mahatma, but if you so desire it, you will be completely linked in. Many times the personality of the individual changes while he is being overshadowed and then goes back to his own personality afterwards. When this happens, the ego must be completely removed.

In the Bible it says, ". . . few saw the Christ that overshadowed Jesus." This is like the overshadowing of the Hierarchy over various individuals in the Teaching. Many people feel this is an imposition and their personality is being taken away. This is not a possession or anything like that, but to be overshadowed by a higher spiritual force is the most wonderful thing that could happen because it brings absolute cosmic wisdom, and this is the only way it can be brought about. It cannot be taught in schools or learned from books. It comes through a development of striving, and as you strive and work through meditation and living ethics you will change yourself, because the Hierarchy never changes anyone. Even the Guru does not have the right to impose good on the disciple. You protect them and pray for them and you hope, but they must do it themselves.

Protection

78. There is a process for living in both the physical or mundane and the Subtle World simultaneously. It's not good to live in an ivory tower and shut the door to the outside world. This helps no one but yourself. The whole idea of a spiritual life is not one of living somewhere in a monastery. You should be in the world but not of it.

When your feet are on the ground and your head is in the Subtle World, then you are working with the creative energies and you become one with this thing of wisdom. The more often you can bring this unity of the two worlds into your daily life and not allow yourself to be touched by anger or hatred or fear, the stronger this bond with the Subtle World becomes and you will have absolute protection.

The Hierarchy says over and over, "Give us your anger, give us your prejudice, give us your grief, give us all these ugly garments and we will give you our shield of protection." If you say, "I have this protection," you have and nothing can touch you.

There is a story about this well dressed man who went down into the subway at Lexington and 58th in New York. He passed a suspicious looking character who was just standing there, so a little farther on he stopped and waited. The next man who came down was very poorly dressed and the suspicious looking man held him up. The one who was well dressed called the police and had him arrested and when they all appeared before the judge he asked the suspect, "Why didn't you hold up this man?" referring to the one more expensively dressed. The robber said, "There were two of them." But there weren't, he only saw two. This was the man's protection.

In Tibet a band of people went to the neighboring village to help bring in the harvest. When it was time to return, they lingered awhile longer because the weather was fine but they stayed too long and when they reached the pass, they found some bandits had cut them off. They were told psychically, "Pull over to the side of the road on your horses with all your equipment but have no fear and do not move." The bandits went right past them. One bandit said, "Look, there are horses and people over there," but the others just laughed and said, "Our crazy friend makes rocks into people."

You too have the protection of the Hiearchy if you have no fear. If you have fear you have no protection. FDR said a very wise thing, "There is nothing to fear but fear itself."

Another example of the protection of the Hiearchy is the story of this chap who came to class about six times in a row and then he went overseas to the war, and when he came back I didn't hear from him for a long time until one day the phone rang and he was terrified. He had left his wallet in a phone booth with four or five hundred dollars in it and theater tickets and everything. I said, "Forget it. Go home and ask for help from the Hierarchy and then in two hours go back to the store and enquire for the manager." He went back in two hours and they had his billfold with all the money and tickets in it. Somebody had turned it in, but they had taken it and then had to bring it back.

Another time there was a fire in this house and everything burned but the books of the Teaching. The same thing happened to J.D. when he was studying with Frank Lloyd Wright. The mice were gnawing on some matches and the whole tent burned during the day while he was away. The only thing that was left was *Fiery World I*. It wasn't even scorched. Everything was gone but the book was untouched.

The little Buddha I have has disappeared three different times. One time I was in Toronto and there were about twenty people at this party. They said, "R., will you show us the Buddha from Tibet?" I said, "Well, I'd rather not," but they said, "Oh come on, be a sport." I said, "Okay," and brought it out and it was passed around and every one looked at it and then I said, "May I have my Buddha back?" and everyone said someone else had it. So I thought, it's fallen into the chair or on the floor and after the party we'll look for it. So we looked and searched and pulled up the edge of the rugs but nothing, it was gone. I said, "Well, I shouldn't have shown it. It was my carelessness for bringing it out."

I was traveling with these cousins of mine and so we packed our bags and took a boat from Toronto to Niagara on the Lake, and when we got there, there were no taxis. Suddenly this car pulled up and this chap said he had been awakened from sleep by a voice that said, "You'd better go to Niagara on the Lake and pick up R., because there are no taxis." I hardly knew this person. On the ride home they were saying, "Too bad you lost your Buddha." I said, "Well, no use crying about it." We walked into the house and into the bedroom I was to use and there on the bed sat my Buddha. We were now about sixty miles from where I had lost it.

The second time this happened we were in San Francisco at a restaurant. Five of us were seated around this table and they begged me on to show the Buddha. I said, "No, the last time I did, I lost it." But they said, "Oh come on, come on." So I said, "Okay, I can't lose it here." As each one was looking at it I kept track of it but suddenly it was gone. We looked on the floor. We called the waiter and I said, "Here is twenty dollars if you can find the little Buddha we lost." Six months later I put on an old pair of painting trousers I hadn't worn for a long time, put my hand in the pocket and there was my Buddha. That's happened three times so now I'm very careful about showing it.

My Buddha was given to me many years ago through the Dalai Lama. They are made of solid gold or silver. Mine is made of silver. They are used in the Tibetan prayer styles. These styles are great big blocks of stone and these little Buddhas are sealed in along with the sacred prayers of Buddha and this acts as a magnet. You find them along the highways as you go into Tibet.

All of these are examples of how precise and total the protection of the Hierarchy is.

79. What is the outer lotus? This is the aura of the guru and is over the disciple for his complete protection. It's the protective net, the impregnable armour.

80. The boys being killed in Viet Nam will be reborn faster and be brought back into better conditions, into better families, with more abilities, with better chances for education—everything. This is the method of helping many people who are not given the chance of doing their thing.

Those who are doing their thing have this great protection which some call luck but it isn't; it's an absolute protection you are born with. But people who have no awareness have nowhere to turn to, are wide open to harm or injury and have no protection.

Brotherhood

81. Many times you will look clairvoyantly at an individual and right here on the forehead is a purple rose. This is a sign of the Brotherhood. In the Teaching they say, "Welcome, reader, for the third time." You have probably been in the Teaching many hundreds of times or you couldn't sit through a session or pick up a book and be able to read it. When you realize we have all been together over and over and over; everytime an Avatar has come, the Brotherhood is brought together for that particular purpose. Many of you were working at the time of Christ and at the time of Buddha. We always come together at those times when we are needed to help bring in a certain Teaching. We have been Jews, we have been Mohammedans, we have been Hindus, we have been everything.

It's like Ramakrishna who had a complete knowledge of Christianity, and Buddhism, Judaism, Zoroastrianism, and Hinduism—this complete knowledge—and he was a man who never went through grammar school, but he had this cosmic or inner wisdom and was able to tap it. Everything is in your subconscious mind and all you have to do is pull it out and utilize it. All your experience, all your wisdom, all your discrimination, all you are today is the sum and substance of what you were from past lives.

82. On the back of the American dollar bill there are two highly mystical symbols, placed there by the Brotherhood. On the left side there is an uncapped pyramid with an "all seeing eye" floating in space. The triangle of the pyramid symbolizes Father, Son and Holy Ghost; Guru, Guide and Master; science, art, and religion. The "all seeing eye" in the apex of the pyramid is also found in the Masonic Order and it signifies the development of the third eye or clairvoyance. When the American people reach that development of spirit which will allow them to see what is beyond the vision of the human eye, and when they become one with complete cosmic consciousness and straight knowledge, the cap will be united with the pyramid, the dollar bill will be redesigned and this will mean the end of Armageddon, the end of the struggle between the forces of dark and light.

On the right side of the bill there is a bird that looks like an eagle, but if you examine it under a magnifying glass, you will see that it is a phoenix. This is the mystical bird that flies into space, drops an egg and then bursts into fire, and a new phoenix arises from the ashes. The egg is the symbol of the spirit and the fire is the fiery energy of creativity.

Out of the ashes of the Old, the New World was created. In the history books, America was always called the New World. A new age was to come to this country where there was freedom of religion and all these various freedoms, and this is why people left the Old World. The old forms of society and politics, etc., have to be reworked into new forms, and this is why America was created.

George Washington and Ben Franklin and many more of our founding fathers were members of the White Brotherhood. This secret Brotherhood has existed from the beginning of time. It's not something far away and mysterious and strange but right here working among men for the service of mankind. These men devoted their lives to the creation of America. They had the courage and daring to sign their names to the Declaration of Independence. They were not thinking of their life and time but of our life and time. The Brotherhood always works for the advancement of science, art, philosophy or in any way to make this a better world. If we can make this a better world for one person we have justified our existence here on earth.

To go back to the dollar bill for a moment: capital punishment is holding back the development of the consciousness of America. Gradually we are breaking down such myths as: no Catholic could become president, or a Jew, and Negroes are becoming mayors and governors, but capital punishment is a violation of a cosmic law and until we abolish this we cannot develop spiritually. Until we work with and accept these true laws of the Ten Commandments, the "all seeing eye" on the dollar bill will continue to float in space.

83. There is a whole new interest now in the life of Origen. When he was eight he had a complete understanding of Christ and Christianity and was teaching in his father's school as a very young boy. In Princeton, New Jersey, they're publishing some books on his philosophy. The Vedanta Center in Los Angeles has his books.

What he did was take the Christianity that Christ taught and the esoteric works of the East and brought it all together just as we are trying to do here. He explained many of the parables that Christ taught through the teachings of Eastern philosophy, but of course it's all one. Many times the mystery of the Bible is hidden, but if you know the key then you know the Bible. As I have often said, "Christ was one of the great esoteric teachers." He went to India and to Tibet and was a member of the Essenes, which is one of the orders of the White Brotherhood.

The Essenes were in existence one hundred years before Christ, one hundred years during the time of Christ and one hundred years after Christ. Then they changed form and became the Knights Templar, and then they became the Meistersingers and then the Night Riders of France and Italy.

The whole purpose of all these Brotherhoods was to fight injustice wherever they found it, even in their own home. Truth was Truth and this was Divine Truth. It was like the English laws that still exist. Whatever crime a man commits, the punishment is the same whether he is a commoner or a Royal Prince. The law is the law for everyone. There is no exception to it. Many people say, "My ethics are for the convenience of the moment," but this is not ethics at all. Your ethics are for twenty-four hours a day and either you're working with it or you're not.

The one great wish of Origen was to be crucified. His father was crucified and every one of his disciples was crucified, but he lived to be about eighty-five and they wouldn't touch him. When he wrote these many wonderful things the Catholic Church made him a saint, but later they threw him out and then they reinstated him and then out again for three times. Now he's in.

84. The Egyptian Freemasonry that Cagliostro was to be head of was actually to be for men, women and children; but this caused a great deal of difficulty with the other Masons, who wanted to eliminate the women and children, and for a long time they did.

Free Masonry was brought out before the French Revolution and it became extremely active. At this time the whole esoteric teaching of the Brotherhood was brought out into the open. The Knights Templar and the Troubadours and all of the initiations are part of the order of the Brotherhood. The Knights Templar are the occult order of Masonry. The plays are written with occult truths and the costumes are made of the finest silks and broadcloths, trimmed with real ermine and sable and they are fantastic. The swords are made of pure silver and gold.

That all began with two men on a white horse. They were so poor they only had one horse, which they used to patrol the path to the tomb of Christ. They protected the Christians, who were making their pilgrimage to Jerusalem, from the Arabs who would attack and rob them. Later it became one of the most powerful orders in all Europe.

Today there are only a very few people in the Scottish Rite that know about the Order of the Brotherhood. I talked to a young man in San Francisco and advised him to go into the Masons knowing what he knows and put this back into Masonry. He said, "R., I've talked to many, many people and they don't know what I'm talking about. The words are all there. It's all there in the plays. They recite the words but there is no meaning."

It's like we were saying about the prayer. If you actually take words of any prayer and think them through as you say them, you will benefit. You will actually experience it. For instance, in the prayer, when you say, "May we link with all outer spaces," the moment you have said this and thought it, you have. That's all it needs. When you say, "The Lord is my shepherd," and feel it, then it is so. You have to take it into your mind and then from the mind into the heart and then you have it—you've got it—it's there!

85. Troubadours are still in existence. They sit cross-legged either in costume or in regular clothes with an unsheathed sword across their knees. This is the symbol of the sword of truth. They either sing or tell stories. The Meistersingers are another form of troubadour. They sing about the beautiful face of the woman they cannot name. This is the Mother of the World.

86. The Druids brought in all the mysteries from England, Ireland and Scotland. They came from the Samothrace in Greece. This island still exists and is part of the White Brotherhood. If you are interested in the Druids there is an excellent book by Talbot Mundy called *Tros of Samothrace.*

87. All the people who are part of the great White Brotherhood

are buried with three red roses in their hand and the casket is never opened. This means they have served their assigned period of time and the body is taken to Shambhala.

When they opened Shakespeare's tomb they found a body with a broken neck which was obviously some man who had been hanged and not his body at all.

As you know, FDR was buried in a sealed casket. I knew his secretary and one day I said to her, "I'd like to ask you a personal question about the last request of FDR." And she said, "Well, if it's not too personal." I said, "Was he buried with three red roses in his hand?" She said, "Yes, but how did you know?" I said, "That's all I want to know because that tells the whole story."

When Rubinstein (Anton, 1829–1894) died just before the (Russian) revolution, he was buried in a sealed casket. Some twenty years later the Bolsheviks came and ripped open the casket looking for jewels, but what they found were three red roses—and they were as fresh as if they had just been placed there—and the body was in a perfect state of preservation.

Guru

88. Guru is the Sanskrit word for teacher. The idea of having a physical teacher is to keep you from getting into difficulty or from getting misinformation. If your teacher is invisible how to do you know it isn't your subconscious mind telling you this is your spiritual teacher? The purpose of the Guru is to instruct you spiritually and to shorten your path as much as possible.

If you are ill or in trouble he will know at once from any distance, and send his thought to help you. Many times a disciple will call and no matter where we are we will hear them. Their call will even awaken us out of a sound sleep. We recognize them by the sound of their voice.

One night in San Francisco I was in a very deep sleep and the voice of a very dear friend of mine, Rose Quan, woke me. I heard her call me three times. It was so clear it woke me up. I immediately telephoned New York and asked one of my disciples to go and see if Rose was all right. They went and found that she had been taken to the hospital that day and at that exact hour they thought she was going to pass. She said to me later, "R., I thought I was dying and I called your name three times." That is how this association works. This woman is not a disciple but a very dear soul in her nineties and we are very *sympatico*. In this great love she has for me and I have for her there is this union, and this union exists among the disciples also.

It is called the "silver cord," and at initiation it comes from the heart of the student and goes right to the heart of the Guru, and that link remains forever unless the student breaks it. No matter where you are, even after death, that cord is there and its purpose is to help and comfort you.

I quote from the Teaching, "Unless you have a physical guru you cannot attain a high spiritual consciousness." You cannot develop beyond a certain point. You can go to church and be very devoted and talk to your priest or rabbi but this does not make you a better person. This is what is expected of you anyway. You should start with that. Then the guidance of the teacher is what takes you beyond.

The Guru, the Guide and the Master; the triangle with the all seeing eye. This is the trinity. Christians call it Father, Son and Holy Spirit. Now when you have the trinity, then you have unity and you have cosmic knowledge. That's the only way you can get it. Only one man, Socrates, did it without a guru.

The Guide does not speak words to you, but as you are working with your Mahatma and your Guru, you may have the same experience some of my disciples have had. Many times they would write a letter and say this was my question and this is what you told me the moment I wrote it. This is the answer. Is this correct? And it is. So this happens when you are utilizing that link (with the Guru) for cosmic or straight knowledge, and you can tune in and use it at any time. That's the whole idea of it, and then you link from there to the Mahatma.

When you attain a certain development, a Mahatma will appear and give you instructions. They won't appear every day or every five minutes, and they don't tell you how wonderful you are, but they will give you exactly what you need to help someone else. Your own things you work out yourself. For instance, when I have a problem with a student or disciple that I don't know how to solve I take it to Roerich and say, "What am I to do, tell me?" and he tells me. It's a verbal voice speaking just like mine is speaking to you and it's short and snappy and right to the point. They don't waste five minutes and they don't waste words.

89. Each person's approach to God is extremely individual, and although we are all working together we are doing it in our own particular way; therefore, each one has to work out their own solutions. Some have a great deal depending on their striving and

devotion. Actually the whole key to it is that link between Guru and disciple because the stronger that link is the more you're going to get out of it and the more the teacher will open your potential if you will allow it. The whole purpose of the Guru is to bring you to the feet of your Master and do this more speedily without error or mistakes. In the first place, any disciple would have to have a potential or he wouldn't be one. It's like a great chain. Here is the Master, here is the Guru and here is the disciple and They are intertwined and neither one can be bypassed.

Many times a disciple feels he wants to go off on his own and not work with the teacher completely. There's no use having one in that case because that's what the teacher is for, to help you avoid making mistakes, and the moment you cut yourself off you cut off your development and there you remain.

Like my communication with my teacher: even though he is gone, when I need his advice that link is so strong I get it immediately. So as you strengthen that bond between Guru and disciple it becomes like a rope and the whole idea is to be able to communicate after death, but this won't happen if you go off on your own and say, "I'm going to do this my way." It's not that you are not allowed to do what you want—anyone can do what they want—but they can also make terrible mistakes and in so doing can cut off the link. I don't mean permanently but it's like having a telephone and not using it. Many times people say, don't bother the teacher by calling him because he's busy, but this is the thing that sets them off in limbo and they go ahead and do their own thing and this is a great mistake.

90. Some people in the Teaching make an excuse not to tell the Guru everything because they say the Guru is clairvoyant. This is because they are afraid he will tell them what is wrong and they don't want to hear that. And sometimes this will happen with the disciples. They say, "You have to get off on your own and do your own thing." This is the idea that you can do what you want and feel justified.

Unfortunately you can't do that. You have to play it straight. You can't kid yourself, and if you try, you don't hurt anyone but yourself. To avoid the Guru is to avoid responsibility. The minute you start that your ego is involved and away you go.

91. When you have made your relationship with your Guru a commonplace thing, then you have lost it.

My clairvoyance was given to me by the Hierarchy to help people avoid making a mistake. That's the whole purpose of the Guru. He can advance the disciple through three or more lifetimes if he will listen to the Guru. There is an actual pattern to the lifetimes of the disciples and many of them know their future lives. There are definite qualities that have to be attained in a certain order. But you cannot regress. What you have gained you will have, even though you may not use it in the next lifetime. Cycles are devoted to attaining a certain quality in every lifetime, for once you start on an ascending spiral you keep on ascending, you don't stop.

92. You should think of your Guru as a very real person. This is how I feel about my Guru. He is alive and right with me all the time. I think of him constantly. I speak to him silently and we are together completely. You can bring about that unity by having a great love and devotion for him. The more love you have the easier it is to contact him.

On the subject of love for the teacher, I have these two very dear friends of mine, both medical doctors and very intellectual and very successful and wealthy. Both had had wonderful healings and later on they went to India. While they were away I got it in meditation one day that they had met their Guru. So I was very happy for them and when they came back, they invited me to dinner. I said, "You met your Guru. I know." They said, "Wellll yessss." I said, "This is a tremendous thing. What do you mean yessss? Did you ask him for initiation?" "Well, noooo." "Why not? This is the most wonderful opportunity in your life. You've wanted it all your life. You've talked about it. Why not?" "Well," they said, "His disciples would kiss his feet." I said, "Did he ask you to kiss his feet?" and they said, "Noooo he didn't, but his feet were dirty."

Oh, for God's sake! I was really disgusted. This is lightmindedness. Here they had in the palm of their hand something terrific and they threw it away. They'll probably not get another chance for four or five lifetimes. Both men are brilliant people with degrees a mile long behind their names but they have no heart. This was their difficulty. They were afraid. Their egos were afraid to let go so the dirty feet was their excuse. If they could only have kindled that heart quality they could have reached the top in this lifetime. They both had good possibilities but they were too intellectual.

93. The Guru always works for the benefit of his disciples, always! Paul Brunton's Guru was Ramahara Maharshi who lived in India. He wanted to go back to see him before his death but instead he went to England and the Maharshi died.

Now this is a very special thing that happens when the Guru is dying. Usually the disciples come and receive a special blessing. This is the most tremendous thing in the world. There is nothing greater, because by this special blessing you make your link with the Guru that much stronger.

The Hierarchy is a unified organization working to help the

consciousness of mankind, and every person who is seeking and looking and working and striving sincerely is under Their guidance and benevolent protection. They are interested in every individual. They are going to watch over each one and protect them and take care of them because those who are seeking do not exist in thousands but in tens.

There is a wonderful saying that no matter where you are— whether it be in the middle of the desert or on the top of a mountain or in Timbuktu—when you are ready, the Guru appears. The timing is always perfect.

The disciple tends to reincarnate when the Guru does. Sometimes they will skip an incarnation because of special work to do but the stronger you forge that link and hold that link with love and devotion the closer you will become with your Guru and the more you will benefit.

Devotion to the Guru is not to his personality, but is to the ideal of the Guru. Roerich had a beautiful story. He saw this boy on the beach and the sun was rising and he said to the boy, "Look at the sun rising," and the boy said, "Yes, it's a beautiful sun." Roerich said, "When you found your Guru was it like the rising of the sun?" and the boy said, "No, sir, it was like seven suns."

If someone approaches me and asks if I am their Guru I have to say no, because if they don't know then they aren't ready. You must know it in your own heart. Like when I met my Teacher, I said, "You are my Teacher and I want to be your disciple." He said, "How do you know?" And I said, "With every pore of my body, every nerve, every muscle, every thought." Always when you are ready the Guru will appear.

94. Patience is one of the great things in our development. Roerich had a little trick of handing you a ball of string that was all twisted and matted. He would say, "Undo it." From this I learned many a lesson in patience, because patience was one of the things I did not have. I unravelled many balls of string.

95. A talisman that is given to the disciple by the Guru should be buried with the disciple when he dies because it has a special spiritual nature to it. You never give away what your guru has given you unless he tells you to give it away and gives you another one. For instance, I've been told to loan mine to other people. I've had two or three talismans. However, the bead stays with the disciple always.

96. Roerich's Guru is Kuinji and I use his name in my prayer because it brings me closer to him. Through one of my disciples introducing me to Kuinji's paintings, I feel a very strong link and in

my own paintings there is a strong influence of Roerich's Teacher. We paint in the same key.

Kuinji was a great, great soul with great kindness, great consideration and great, great love. Roerich had a studio five flights up and one day Kuinji came to criticize his paintings. By this time he was an old man but he walked all the way up and criticized his work and then he walked all the way down. But then he felt maybe he had been too severe and so he walked all the way up the five flights to tell him, "I didn't mean to be so severe but I love you and I want you to be a great artist."

This is one of the great things of Mahatmaship, this consideration of other people. It's the whole thing. Not consideration of oneself but of others.

97. An Ashram is any place where there is a Guru. It's usually a place where students may come, a place for men, women and children, because they all have equal rights to God consciousness.

In the old days in many of the Moslem churches only the men were allowed in the church and the women had to stay home. In the Greek churches the men stand on one side and the women on the other and in the early Christian period around 555 A.D. the women were not supposed to have a soul, and they had gems like that in their doctrine, but in the New Age there is no sex. A soul is sexless. If a man, woman or child is striving, their spirit is developing and this is what creates the soul and that's the important thing.

Every Ashram and every group that is working occultly is penetrating out into space to the other planets, and they are penetrating in. This is why they say in *The Call, (Leaves of Morya's Garden I)* every Ashram is a light that reaches out into infinity. It works both ways. The more light there is on Earth to penetrate out, the more benevolent rays can come. With all the New Agers coming in there will be more and more groups of Yogis.

Guide

98. Everyone has a separate and personal Guide given to them at birth for one lifetime. As we develop and evolve so does our Guide. At death it stays with you through Devachan and then leaves and attaches itself to somebody else.

The Guide never becomes a human form. It's a devic form. A deva is a spirit without a body. The Guide is your conscience or basic part of your intuition. This is part of the trinity within us. It's always Guru, Guide and Master, or Father, Son and Holy Ghost, the trinity.

This is a very, very important thing. When you become a Mahatma you will have lifted the Guide to that development and then it leaves and goes on to another person. The Mahatma no longer needs the Guide because He has become master of Self. It is at this time He becomes immortal. When the child is born, it's the mother and father who have attracted the quality of that child by their development. Then this high consciousness of the Guide will come into the child like a beautiful gift. The Guide and Guardian Angel are one and the same thing.

This is the thing that tells you, don't take that plane or don't get on that lift. I had an experience in New York in one of the department stores. I stood in front of the elevator and it was just as if I were frozen. I could not move. People pushed around me and gave me dirty looks but I was powerless to move. The other people got into the elevator and went up to the sixth floor and down it came. A lot of people were injured. Of course when this happened I was near a phone, called an ambulance and got help.

The more you listen the more your Guide will help you. It's a very personal thing. I remember the picture, "Mr. Deeds Goes to Washington," with Jimmy Stewart. The story was about his Guardian Angel who was a real bungler. He bungled everything until Jimmy Stewart said, "I wish you'd go away." He'd say, "I can't. I can't." It was very funny.

Many people mistake the Guide for the teacher, but it's not, it's your intuition. If you develop and listen to a very fine Guide, this is splendid, but it's not the ultimate because it's only to guide you until you come to a place where you take an image that will take you beyond that. The Guide can only go so far.

Disciples and Discipleship

99. There is an esoteric law that says if you study any religion or philosophy for two years you have earned the right to ask for discipleship.

This is what was meant when Christ said, "... men twice born, born of the flesh and born of the spirit." Born of the spirit means initiation, just as Jesus was initiated by John the Baptist who was his Guru. The same form is still used today. It's an old Hindu method of using holy water from the Ganges, and fire and incense and sound and flowers.

The Christian baptism is a dissipation of the old form of initiation in which they immerse the whole body in a tank of water. Of course, the Catholic and Episcopal churches have flowers on the altar and burn incense, and there are temple bells in most churches. The symbols are there but the meaning is gone.

So, at the end of two years you have earned the right for probation and from the moment you start your probation the Mahatmas turn a battery of lights upon every action, every thought, and every deed. They will be watching you twenty-four hours a day and when you have passed Their tests, They will tell your Guru and he will tell you the month, the day, and the hour of your initiation. The length of probation can be any amount of time depending only on you.

Every three years there is a special test. This is true of students as well as probationaries and disciples. If you fail the test you must wait another three to seven years until you are given another chance to prove yourself. In the meantime your development is temporarily arrested.

100. Discipleship means that at the moment of initiation a silver cord comes out from the heart of the Guru to the heart of the disciple and attaches itself at that moment. Some people see it and some don't, but nearly everyone feels it. This link is forever unless the disciple breaks it. The teacher can never break it, and as a disciple grows in love and devotion that cord becomes like a rope and this link remains beyond life, beyond death or any place in the world. That's why they call it the silver cord.

At initiation the aura of the Guru covers the aura of the disciple and this is called the double protective net and no dark force can penetrate it. Only the disciple can break it and when this happens, it's like a kick in the stomach and you are ill for two or three days. Then there is a hole in the aura and obsession can come in. That is why we warn you, do not jump into discipleship until you know what you are doing.

There is an exact moment of breaking that link between the disciple and Guru. It can be broken with the thought, "Oh why did I get into this?" It's a very delicate thing. Just one thought like that and it's gone. If the link is very strong with devotion maybe one thought wouldn't break it, but two or three would. When Peter denied Jesus three times, that's what happened.

An example of this is F. He began to find fault with the Teaching and said he wanted something else and he was dissatisfied, and just like that in five minutes it was gone. The three boys who have broken are back now as students. They are very fine people and I love them very much but they have broken and they know this and they cannot have that relationship again in this lifetime. For one of them Master M. said, "You must take the cord your bead was on and knot it up and wear it on another cord as a constant reminder of what you have done." Having doubts or second thoughts about the Teaching is one violation that cannot be made and this is why they say, be sure, be very sure you know what you are doing. It's a tremendous responsibility and it's not easy. It's blood, sweat and tears. If anything breaks your confidence or faith in the Teaching, it's gone.

You see, at initiation it's two souls suddenly being wedded together in spirit. It's a marriage of spirits that's forever, and the minute there is regret or you feel cramped or this is not for you that silver cord is broken. This is why they call it the unseen gift because you can carry it into eternity or you can smash it to pieces.

101. When a disciple has gone fifteen or twenty years and then breaks, a new co-worker is sent and all the experience of the one who broke is given to him. This never fails to happen and is done so that nothing is wasted.

In India there was this man who meditated in this one spot under this tree for twenty years and nothing happened. He didn't attain Samadhi, so he got up and left. A wandering tramp came by and saw this place and he said to himself, "Ah, somebody has been meditating. I think I'll try it." So he sat down and just like that he attained enlightenment. Had the other man meditated just one more day he would have had it. His twenty years were given to another person in one flash. You see, it was impatience. This is why many persons lose out by just an hour or a day.

When someone breaks, they lose the protection of the Hierarchy that was given to them when they became a disciple. The double aura from the Guru to the disciple is torn away and in that tear obsession can come in and this is the danger.

Of course in the next incarnation they can come back. The Teaching says, "If not in this lifetime, then in the next or the next or the next." The idea is that you can finish all your karma in this one lifetime, but the Teaching comes to you in many lifetimes.

We have been everywhere, done everything, been everything. We've been colored, Jewish, Chinese—we've been everything. Being in this Teaching means we have lived many thousands and thousands of lives.

This is why they say Mahatmas are made on this Earth and on no other planet. There are less than one hundred Mahatmas in our solar system, so it's not easy. It can be done in seven years but it means complete selflessness. That and healing are the fastest ways of development. When we can put others ahead of ourselves or take pain away from other people, it speeds up our whole development. What greater thing can you do than take away someone's pain and agony?

102. All initiates have come from another planet like Venus or Jupiter and did not go through transmigration here on Earth. They actually descended to Earth and took an envelope from the Earth people and were born as an Earth child but with the consciousness of their own planet. The fact that by their sacrifice they came to Earth is their good karma, because they are here to raise the consciousness of humanity and in so doing they are adding to their own development.

103. There are various ways that you are being taught as a disciple. Some are taught by lips to the ear, some by action, some by performance, some by suggestion, some by the heart, and some by silence. So there is not one way on that spiral of development but many ways. The more advanced a disciple becomes the more he is taught intuitively. Like the holy man we met the other day: there was a tremendous power of suggestion in his presence.

104. Discipleship goes on and on and up and up. It's a continuous thing. I had a letter recently from one of my disciples in New Mexico in which she said, "I am preparing now for my next life. I want to find my Guru very early when I am young." This is a very wonderful thing to strive for.

I have had people on their deathbed say, "I know I haven't made it in this lifetime but in my next life will you accept me?" This is a beautiful thing because the contact is made and it's not nonsense at all. It's really a thing of planning.

105. One of the things they stress in the Teaching is that a disciple or pilgrim on the path must produce creatively. This creative thing is very important to their development; otherwise they just stagnate and accumulate knowledge. But if you work in any creative field that is open to you, this will speed up your whole development. This is why many of our people are painters, engineers, scientists, etc., all working with these creative forces and this speeds up their whole evolution.

106. The greatest impediment to spiritual growth in a disciple is first of all spiritual pride. Ego is another. Contentment is another, and also being satisfied. In the East they constantly tell you, divine dissatisfaction with yourself is the most wonderful and healthy way to develop.

When you can say, I'm lazy, I'm shirking my job and I'm going to do something about it, this is very good because you're throwing off an old garment.

Or you may say, I've been stealing other people's ideas and I'm going to stop it. In one of my classes I suggested they make a list of all the good things about themselves and then make a list of bad things and work on it. So this young chap brought me his list and he said, "I'm a thief," and I said, "You're not a thief. This I know about you." He said, "Yes, I am. I steal other people's ideas and that's just as bad as if I stole money, and I'm going to stop it." This is absolute honesty. If we can work with this kind of honesty within ourselves, then we can be false to no one.

As I've often said, Agni Yoga is a game and to play it you have to be absolutely honest with yourself. You can't kid yourself. You have to be able to say I have this fault or that fault, I'm not proud of it but I recognize it and I'm going to do something about it. Many people say, I told a white lie, but it's still a lie. They play these games and it's very bad. Be very critical and ask yourself, "Am I adjusting to conditions just to be pleasant or is this dishonest?"

When I was a decorator I went into this beautiful home which had obviously been done by an excellent decorator. I said to the lady, "Your home is beautiful," and she said, "Thank you, I did it myself." I knew she hadn't and then she looked at me and said, "I'm sorry, I didn't do it myself as you very well know. It was done by Sloans but my ego wanted you to think I had done it." It's in little ways like this that we play games with our honesty. Don't do it.

Another thing we have to watch out for is competition. There are no two people with the same development and no two people who are alike. Everyone is entirely individual. The more diversified the people are the better. This is one of the great things about the people in the Teaching. Believe me they are diversified. They are all strong individuals and this is very good. When you can take all these souls and blend them together to become one with the whole Source, then you have the key. This is what is meant when we use the prayer, "The dewdrop slips into the blue green sea." The soul is the drop of water. The sea is God and we are all one with that. Once your drop of water is in the sea you can't take it out. It's all one.

It's really very simple when you go right to the point of what is Truth and say I'm going to play this game honestly; these are my faults, I'm going to be aware of them and get rid of them. If you're not aware of them, you'll never get rid of them.

If your spirit is functioning in its true place by being one with the Divine Source, then you are in perfect balance. If you're not, then you're out of balance and this is why people have difficulties, why the unhappiness, why the groping for things, the seeking to understand.

Now, when you can bring your spirit into equilibrium and have this unity within yourself, then you have happy people who have this completeness within.

Only the spirit can develop the soul. Only the spirit can do this, so if it's not functioning as it should in light or illumination or wisdom then it's out of balance because its function is to bring joy, joy, joy into your life. As They say in the Teachings, "If your religion or philosophy does not bring you joy, then it doesn't fit you." That joy they speak of is the balance or equilibrium of the spirit. The personality is that part of the soul that involves the ego. It's the emotions that cause complications and throw the whole thing off balance. The soul is more gross but the spirit is absolutely pure and when we can achieve this perfect balance then we have the twin soul developed in the one person. Then we have the synthesis that makes Mahatmaship.

107. One of my students asked: "In one of the books of the Teaching we read that even terror was good as long as there was no fear, but we can't see how you can be terrified without being afraid."

You might be terrified by seeing a Mahatma but you would have no fear. You may be terrified of what He can read in your mind or see in your aura.

Or, for instance, when a disciple comes to me and says, "I am terrified for fear I will lose my discipleship," that terror is very excellent because if you can think that way you're on the edge of the abyss and you'll never fall off. You'll always stay right there. But if you say, "I'm getting along fine, I've nothing to worry about," watch out. You should even be terrified of what the reaction might be to your thinking because that link can be broken with a thought, the thread is so delicate. So, one walks softly.

The more terror you have of losing something precious the less likely you are to lose it, but if you have no concern it may slip away very easily. It's not when the going is rough that you need worry, but when the going is easy; that's when you are liable to lose the very thing you want most. This is often true of people who come into the Teaching; if they have experienced great hardships or sadness or great difficulties with their health, they come for that reason. But people whose health is fine and who have a great deal of money and are having a good time have no need for God. It's only when you reach a great crisis that there is a great need and void and then you do something about it, so it pays to be a little terrified.

108. Buddha tested his disciples by telling them to go out and bring back the most precious thing they could find. Some brought back jewels, some brought great precious paintings and some brought

a flower because it has given its life to bring beauty into the world.

Another test was to bring a tray containing many things with a napkin over it. He would raise the napkin for a few seconds and then lower it and ask them to describe what was on the tray. This was an exercise to sharpen their observation.

109. Very often the question is asked, "What are the seven vegetable oils mentioned in the books of the Teaching?" This is part of the elixir that Count St. Germain gave. Immediately on reading this the student wants to know exactly what it is.

This cannot be given out until the disciple has reached a certain stage of development in his own spiritual consciousness, and only then is it given to them directly by the Mahatma.

This emulsion is made up of common vegetable oils but it's the method of combining them and the way that they are used that's very important to the whole physical body. It revitalizes the body from old age.

There's another thing that the American Indians have, called joe-pye weed. I asked an old Indian out in Taos, New Mexico, about this and he said, "Have you ever seen an old Indian?" and I said, "No." Of course, they were very evasive. They brew it into a tea and drink it. Actually, you never see a very old Indian unless they're drinking whiskey.

Initiation

110. The idea of initiation means that you are opening a whole new door of consciousness.

Initiations have nothing to do with ritual. When the initiate has assimilated the higher rays, then it takes place. If the individual was not ready and you gave them initiation they wouldn't feel anything, nothing would happen, but you see, at initiation something does happen. It changes the individual completely.

The time and place is given by the Mahatmas. It may be in a simple place, in the home, any place, but never in public, never! The only way you can come to initiation is by assimilation of these higher rays, but what you do with it afterwards is up to you. You can go very far or remain right on that level. This is why there are a number of initiations, seven to be exact.

111. I have been asked the question, "When can you begin taking disciples?" When the complete fourth initiation takes place. It's in two parts. I am permitted to tell you the first part, but the second part is between you and your Guru and cannot be revealed.

You will be awakened in the middle of the night; it always happens in the night. The room is pitch black and you will see a silver rose glowing in the darkness. The darkness recedes and the rose glows. You see every leaf, the thorns, the petals. It's like a silver rose of light; a very beautiful thing.

The second part of the fourth you must witness and then you take it to the teacher, the Guru, who listens to your second part and then reads you his second part and it's exactly word for word the same. Then you know the individual has had his second part.

The rose appears and dissolves, but the second part is told and is never put in writing or any book form but is told by the teacher to the disciple and it's forbidden to tell it to anyone else.

In each incarnation you have to go through each initiation all over again until you reach the seventh and then you don't have to do it anymore.

At your fourth initiation, when it is complete, your teacher takes you through the initiations and takes you through your first disciple, and from then on you refer all your disciples to your Guru so you don't make any mistakes, and this saves you a lot of heartaches and the whole thing works out beautifully.

112. Alchemy is turning base metals into gold, and by changing our chemistry through striving we change the grossness of our bodies into the gold of pure spirit.

When we came here from the higher planets millions of years ago to help raise the consciousness of humanity, it was necessary to go through the earthly experience, because if we remembered the fine quality and essence and light we had on the other planet, we would go absolutely mad with the impatience, the stupidity, the blundering of this earth life. Who would you talk to? You wouldn't fit into any society. So it's veiled from you until you begin to develop and then the veils fall away.

That is why the fourth initiation is called the initiation of Isis. Isis is always veiled. This is the beginning of tearing away the veils of maya after which you are able to see directly. This is the beginning of Straight Knowledge. It doesn't mean you have full and complete knowledge, but when you have completed the fourth you have access to Straight Knowledge or the Fiery World. This is why wisdom is so important, as it's all tied up with cosmic knowledge and cosmology. Straight Knowledge is never erroneous. After the fourth then the fifth and sixth initiations are on this plane by your Guru and the seventh is by the Mahatmas. When that happens you are ready to become a Mahatma.

Initiation takes place to everyone alike regardless of their path or religion.

When the disciple receives the fourth completely, the teacher can then teach him the whole initiation which is always done in secret, never written down. Then the new Guru is on his own, except he can bring his disciples to his own Guru for a reading and thereby save himself a lot of headaches. He can tell him how far they can go, what he can do with them, how much he can work with them and where he has to wait and let the student develop on his own.

You cannot force a flower or you will ruin it. The flower has to blossom in its own time, to its own beauty and maturity and development. You can water it and take care of it and see that it is not killed by weeds and that there is not too much force put upon it. This is the idea of *Leaves of Morya's Garden*. We are the gardeners and the people are the flowers in the garden.

There was a man in Cuba, a cousin of Dr. G., who had a very bad illness and we were able to help him and clear it up. Evidently, he was very close to the Hierarchy.

He told me, "You know R., I had this dream one night in which one of the Mahatmas came and took me up the mountain side and this man with a turban was building a garden in miniature. It was the most beautiful and exquisite thing I have ever seen. There were archways and gravel paths and trees and everything was in miniature. I stood there watching while he was working with these rakes and trowels until I got embarrassed. Finally I said, 'Well, I can be a gardener, too.' "

And he told me, "The man turned and it was Morya, and I'll never forget the look he gave me. And he said, 'Well, why don't you?' With that he went right back to his work."

Evidently it was a prophesy. The Cuban had great ability and could have done many wonderful things because his development was tremendous, but he just didn't do it. He was a very wealthy man and got pulled away by too much money and worldly pleasures.

This actually was his chance to do a terrific work, because at that time in Cuba Castro was not yet in power and they were having a lot of trouble with poor diet. He came to me and asked what he could do to help and I told him, "Start a milk fund for all the different schools all over Cuba. You can afford it, and that alone would be a tremendous help."

Well, he didn't follow through on it, and Castro came in and took all his banks and all his money and cleaned him out. Had he done this he would have been a hero and he probably would have gotten out of Cuba with all his money. Instead, he was hanging onto his money and he lost it. It was a very clear cut dream and he was told exactly what to do. The Hierarchy will only tell you once, but, of course, you don't have to do it.

113. In the Teaching they speak of the fiery baptism. This refers to your seventh initiation when you are taken up to 10,000 feet and are taught to handle the fires of space. This is your initiation into Mahatmaship. The Teaching tells you that you can have no drugs, no alcohol, no meat, no impurities for at least two years prior to this or you would be burned to ash.

When you get to this point you are working in a completely different evolution. In your spiritual development you are like the alchemist who turns base metals into gold. As you develop, your chemistry changes. Certain things fall away. Smoking and drinking and various habits fall away. Things like hunger and cold fall away until finally you're completely free.

When you are ready for this fiery baptism you are physically taken above 10,000 feet. You are told to go at a certain time— exactly when, where and how. If you want to do it, fine. If you don't, you can sit for another seven years before you get another chance.

I recommend you read *Zanoni* by Bulwer-Lytton. It's the story of a man who had all these powers and became enamored and lost it all.

114. Everyone has an aura and in the aura there is a symbol about the size of a luncheon plate. It's flat and it may be above the head or it may tilt; it may be to one side or in the back, and this gives you the information of what initiations that individual has had in former lives. For instance, the symbol that is visible at the back and top of the head is the initiation of Isis from an old Egyptian mystery school. It's part of the seed of the spirit, so it's always there.

This is why a Guru is supposed to be clairvoyant: so he can look at the aura of the individual and see if they have been initiated or not, because they can't have two Gurus in one lifetime.

There is a wonderful story in the East about four brothers. Three of the brothers found their Guru and the fourth brother found his Guru, but also took the Gurus of his three brothers. It was fine except when they were going to teach him to fly through the air. The three brothers were given a blast by their Gurus and of course each of them flew. When it came time for the fourth one to fly, all four Gurus gave him a blast and blew him apart.

You see, that's not how it works. You must work with one person only and that person is responsible for you and your development. That's the only way it can operate.

The symbol takes away any guess work or imagination. There it is plain and clear, no mistake.

Spiritual Family

115. Each time an Avatar comes to Earth this beautiful spiritual family comes back to work together and prepare the way for His coming. My disciples have probably been working on this planet for a whole manvantara. They came before Buddha, before Christ, before Zoroaster, and now they are here again to do this special work before the coming of the Maitreya. From the beginning of time there have always been the forerunners, the New Agers who have come to prepare the way.

The bond of our spirits has brought us together. Many times you don't know it's happening or you may get a hint of something, but you can see this tapestry being woven back and forth. You may be asked to do something but you're not given the whole pattern. It's not all laid out for you, but you must do your part. We are nothing but leaders of groups of people, and the idea is to get diversified people working together in unity and harmony and love. That is the whole key to it. When we can love one another without wanting anything in return, then we have it.

If you remember your Greek mythology—where they stole the fire from the Gods and brought it down—in the same way these souls from other planets have come to Earth to lift the consciousness of man because he has potential of mind and development. This is done through culture, and this is why the whole essence of Agni Yoga is beauty, culture and creativeness—all of these things.

In America we are getting more and more music, more and more ballet, more and greater theater, more painting, more of everything. The potential is becoming greater. There are new mediums to work in, new forms, new methods of teaching, new approaches in education, in politics, in everything. There is no limit. Everything is opening up: the sciences and art and religion. And this is developing the mental body as well as the consciousness; not only for the people who are doing it but also for those who can't or won't.

This great enthusiasm is like a fire that's sweeping over a wheat field that's ripe and dry. You can't fight it. Like the little sixteen-year-old girl who brought a drawing to class in New York one night and I said, "Dear, your drawing is beautiful. Your color is lovely." The next month when I was in New York again she had sixteen beautiful drawings. I said, "These are beautiful. Have you been studying?" and she said, "No, you believed in me." There are many people who unknowingly have this spark within them.

116. The Brotherhood exists in both the mundane and the Subtle Worlds, and when you can dwell in both worlds at the same time then you have achieved a balance in your life. When we speak of the Brotherhood we are referring to the Brotherhood of the Hierarchy, and when we are related to each other by a consciousness of the Hierarchy, then we have a true relationship of spirit from seed to seed to seed of spirit, from lifetime to lifetime to lifetime.

This is why the Brotherhood of the Hierarchy exists; whereas the Brotherhood of Freemasons also exists in the Subtle World, but very few Masons know of this binding spirit that brings you together from lifetime to lifetime. Nor do they know that the Hierarchy is the cement that binds this Brotherhood together from as far back as perhaps fifty thousand years, and each time an Avatar has come this Brotherhood has existed and worked together. This is the true spiritual relationship and your family relationship is only karma. This spiritual relationship is beyond karma.

Most families are karmically brought together to work out something from another lifetime. This is why we will have conflicts in our particular families until such time as we can straighten out this karma.

For instance, this young man came to me and wanted to become a disciple and I said, "Look, A., before you can do this you have to go to your stepmother and ask her forgiveness for all the trials and tribulations you have caused her, because you have caused her a great deal of heartache and misery. You have all this resentment toward her because your father told you your mother ran off and left you."

She was with the Imperial Government in Russia, and she was called back to work against the Bolsheviks (1930) and was shot. Instead of telling him the truth, his father said she went off and left him and this left a big, deep scar so that he thought all women were going to betray him. So, with every woman he met, including his stepmother, he would inflict this whole karmic pattern out of fear of being betrayed.

I said, "The only way I can take you as a disciple is if you go home and thank her for all the things she has done for you between the ages of two and twenty-three (the age he was when he came to me) and call her 'mother' and really mean it in your heart. Bring her flowers and candy and sit down and open your heart to her. I'm not asking you to make her into a saint, which she is not, but I am asking you to love her in spite of all her inadequacies, and then you will be released from all this karma."

He said, "Oh, I can't do it. I can't do it." I said, "That is the price of discipleship. When you can do it, fine." Finally, he did it and he came to me and said, "When I sat down and talked to her, all my resentment left me. She broke down into tears and almost died of shock, and suddenly I saw the karma and understood it. I saw that I had given her karma, too, and so we worked it out." This whole karmic relationship just fell apart and spread out like dew upon the grass, and from that moment on they have had a very wonderful relationship.

There are kings of spirit and kings of the Earth, but the most important thing is to be a king of spirit. If you are hurt or insulted, say, "This is only my karma," and if it affects you there is something in you that shouldn't be there. You should be completely impersonal, and when you have conquered that, you have the key to life and life is a ball. But if you harbor resentment toward your family or blame them for things, this is no good. Say, "Okay, this is a karmic debt and I am willing to pay it and pay it gladly;" then it's finished and you're through with it.

As Buddha said, we are on this Wheel of Life, ill fed, well fed, ill housed, well housed and we do not drop from the Wheel until we know what our karma is; what we have to learn from being born into that family.

For instance, this sixteen-year-old girl has a mother who is always drunk. Instead of hating her mother she can try to see what happened to her to bring about this condition. She won't blame her mother but will look at her and say, "This I will try to avoid doing." If she hates her mother and calls her a drunken bitch, she will have to come back to this same situation over and over again until she learns to release it.

A highly evolved spirit can look ahead into their next life and see where they will be reborn and what will happen to them, and who their mothers and fathers will be. It's a perfect karma because they can choose a family that will provide what is needed to make them a more complete person. For instance, they may have all the other attributes—intellectual, etc.—but lack a beautiful heart quality, so they will choose a musical family to be born into and through that relationship learn how this beautiful thing of music can lift the consciousness.

The Guru also arranges for you to be born into a family who can teach you a lesson you need to learn. Sometimes the lesson is not very nice, but you have earned the karma of being placed in that situation and there is no one to blame but yourself. As you sow, so shall you reap.

Many times a family will pull together financially but will destroy each other by criticism. One time I had given A. a job of decorating some buildings. His father called and said, "My boy never finishes what he starts, and I hear he is going to work for you. I wanted to warn you he will never finish the job." I said, "It's very kind of you to call, but I believe in your boy, even if you don't, and he will finish the job." He was a well-intentioned father, but this was a very poor attitude to have toward his child.

There was this boy being taught by Socrates who said, "My mother and father love me very much." Socrates said, "Fine, splendid, but I'll prove to you they don't." He said, "You have a slave at home who is your tutor and your father has made you swear obedience to a slave. This is very undignified. It makes you lower than a slave. You have a chariot driver who drives your horses. Your father doesn't trust you but he trusts a stranger and pays him . . ."

There is a fine line here, because if you really love your children you have absolute faith and trust in them. This goes back to the thing we have spoken of so often: if one person believes in you, you can accomplish anything. You only need one person who really believes in you. It's a constant power.

Many times I've heard mothers and fathers berate their children. Many parents don't love their children. Many have been unplanned, but even if they are planned, the child cries and is a constant responsibility and the parents resent this. They can't travel and they have little or no freedom, and often they take out their frustration on the children by beating them, and yet they will say, "I love my child."

An example of a real parent was the story of this young girl, the daughter of an engineer, who was going around with this boy who was no good and she got pregnant. Instead of the father saying, "Never darken my door again," he said, "Have the child, but for God's sake don't marry the boy or you'll be unhappy the rest of your life. We'll raise the child and give it love and take care of it and do everything we can for it." Now, there was a real father, but how many parents are that way? Most of them get emotional and dictatorial.

This thing of being understanding is all tied up with karma and how unselfish you are. If you really love someone you are completely unselfish about the individual and will sacrifice yourself for their happiness. This is why the Teaching says over and over again, selflessness! Elimination of ego is selflessness. Only when you think of other people are you not thinking of self.

Children

117. New Age children are recognized by their transparent skin, their extremely delicate and fine bone structure, by markings on the hand, and they have the ability to read upside-down without any practice—or down to up—and can do things with both hands. They have a clear perception of color and are attuned to music. They have graceful and beautiful voices, and if you will notice, there is a quality of light coming out of their face and hands. They are extremely intuitive and you cannot lie to them; they know at once.

Frank Lloyd Wright, Nikola Tesla, George Washington Carver, Fisk, Henry Ford, Burbank, Edison were all New Agers. They came in more than one hundred years ahead of their time to help speed up the whole evolution. That was their job. Every year this group of men would get together up in Canada for two weeks on a stated hunting trip, but they always went without guns. They would pool their ideas and pray and meditate together and come away inspired with new creative ideas. The Mahatmas and Rishis are throwing out all these ideas, and these people are putting them into operation.

There are many children aged two to six in the New Age School in Texas who are children of working parents. There are many New Agers among them, just as there are New Agers to be found all over the world. One in every ten thousand is a New Ager.

People from other planets are usually New Agers. If you are working in your true esoteric place, then you are a New Ager. All are highly evolved souls. All have incarnated hundreds of thousands of times. Roerich's job is to bring in all these New Age children, into their proper focus for what they are to be here on Earth.

118. A child has this great awareness of being able to separate the real from the unreal. It is the conditioning that we give him that takes it away. You have to allow the child to function; you have to allow the child to express himself and not be told this is not so, and that doesn't exist, and you mustn't do this, and you mustn't do that.

If a New Age child is born into a family and the family is

chauvinistic and set in their thinking—as for instance, if they are Catholic and think theirs is the only religion and every other religion is wrong—they spoil the quality of the child, unless the child can fight and throw this thing off. This is what has happened to many of these hippies, or flower children; many are New Agers and rejecting these old and useless and antiquated forms and are taking on the new, and in doing so are causing a great deal of trouble among their parents and in the schools and churches.

Now, prejudice starts at the dinner table. Children are taught prejudice. Remember the lines in *South Pacific* where they say, "You have to be taught to learn to hate. You have to be taught to be afraid of people whose eyes are oddly made, you have to be carefully taught." You cannot be born into this world with a dislike for certain people; that's not possible. A child does not know the difference between Chinese or colored or themselves. This is taught by the parents. It's in the home where the potential of the child is damaged by the chauvinism, the prejudice and narrowness of the parents.

There is a wonderful story about children that Lisa Sargio told me one day at lunch. She was on radio station WQXR for a long time and I knew her very well.

She said, "We have this estate out of New York on the river and the children play there. I would go out and tell them, 'Please don't play near the river because it's quite deep and if you fall in we are responsible and I don't want you to drown.' " And she said, "There were two or three colored children playing there also, and I asked them if these were their friends and they said, 'Yes.' I asked, 'Do you play together?' and they said, 'Yes.' And I asked, 'Do you take these children to your home to play?' and they said, 'Oh no, our fathers and mothers wouldn't understand.' "

So this is the way the kids get around it. Whether people are white, green or purple, it doesn't matter, if they are polite and well behaved they are acceptable. It's only when they are raucous, rude and ugly that they're unacceptable, but your discrimination will tell you which it is.

Families are karmic, and we are born into a family for a reason. Maybe it's to learn not to be like some person in the family or maybe it's to be like them. As has been said many times, "We should be an imitation of Christ." If we can be, then we are working in a positive way. We should never condemn our families, but try to understand them.

The child comes in with karma and it is up to the mother and father to help them overcome this karma, and if they can't do this, then the child has to work it out and get rid of it himself.

Sometimes the disciples are placed into a particular family by the teacher to learn a particular lesson. When you have learned that lesson then you will not repeat that same mistake with your children.

What happens to you in this world is nobody's fault but your own. It's not your mother's fault, not your father's fault, not your aunt's or your uncle's. When you can accept the fact that everything in life is karma then you have the answer to the whole thing.

119. The child who has a gift for music will be attracted to a father or mother who also has a gift for music. Many times a very ugly couple will have a child who is perfectly beautiful; in other words, an ugly duckling has hatched a swan. Or, a child will have great refinement and beauty while the parents will be rather crude. The only explanation for this is karma. Then there are children who look exactly like one or the other parent, and children who look nothing at all like anyone in the family.

There is an amusing story about Isadora Duncan, the great dancer, and Bernard Shaw. She sent him a wire and said, "Wouldn't it be wonderful if we had a child with my beauty and your brains." He sent back a wire which said, "Wouldn't it be awful if he had your brains and my beauty."

120. The nerve centers of children can be protected by meditation. All children should be taught meditation, and the earlier the better. At the school in Texas they start at two, three and four years old, and the little ones take to it like ducks to water. They call it "the quiet time."

Many times these youngsters come back and say they remember when they were a dancer or an artist in another life. Many times we come in with these memories, but we're sent to school and Sunday school where we're told there is no such thing as another life; it's all your imagination. The parents and teachers take this from you and ruin it. The child has this native ability to reach back when they are young, but by the time they are seven they begin to lose it by being exposed to the outside world. Meditation keeps this gateway open.

Sometimes children suddenly run very high temperatures for no apparent reason. This is a form of an excess of psychic energy. Watch these children, they are the unusual ones. These are the children of consciousness. If they are sickly when very young, this is a very good sign. The energy is there, but they are unable to control it.

Daydreaming is not a form of meditation. This is not good because you go off into nothing. The idea is to be consciously aware of everything at all times. In the school in Texas they play a game in which there is a tray of various objects and they're covered by a cloth. They lift the cloth for ten or fifteen seconds and then the children are asked to tell what they saw; how many objects, their color, etc. This comes from an ancient system in India where the British Intelligence taught the children to be spies, but it's a good exercise to teach the children to be aware of every thing around them.

121. It's a very good thing to encourage children to ask questions. When I was a very young boy in England, my father had a Danish friend, a wonderful man who was very broad in his concepts. I was making a nuisance of myself with questions and my father told me to shut up and stop asking so many questions. His friend said, "No, don't ever stop. You ask me any question you want and as many as you want at any time, and if I don't know the answer, I'll go and look it up." It was tremendous what he gave me that my own father wouldn't give.

Many times you tell the child to do something and they ask why, and you tell them "because I told you to." This is no answer. You should explain it intelligently and then they will accept it.

You should always talk to children as you would to adults. One day I was talking to a little six-year-old in Los Angeles and he said, "I have an invisible playmate. His name is Richard. Do you believe it?" I said, "Yes, I do, but I don't see Richard." He said, "I don't see him either, but I hear him and he speaks in my ear." I said, "What does he say?" and he went on to tell me some of the things Richard told him and they were not at all childlike. He said, "When I die, Mr. H., will I be invisible like Richard?" and I said, "Yes, very likely." Then he said, "Will the seed of my soul and what is my brain, will I take that with me when I die?"

Now, this is a six-year-old. He had brought this in from another lifetime, but if I had ridiculed him or talked down to him it would have destroyed this beautiful awareness he had. So, always listen to what children have to say and answer them as you would an adult.

122. When a child creates his little playmates off in the corner, people say he has fantasies, but this is not fantasy. This is something quite different. The child is bringing back memories from a past life and these people do exist for that child. This often goes on until they are seven or eight years old and then they lose it.

I just came back from a trip out West, and in Texas there is a little girl, L., who is two and a half. She speaks in full sentences and one day I went into the room where she was playing and I said, "Mishi Hallo," which is a Tibetan greeting. She turned around and said, "Mishi Hallo," perfectly. Now, for a child two years old this is amazing. So, I said two or three other words in Tibetan which she answered perfectly.

I said to her mother, "This is fantastic. Write down everything she says just as it sounds and later on ask her, 'Where are you from and where were you born?' " So a few days later her mother turned to her unexpectedly and said, "Lisa, where did you live before?" and she answered something that sounded like Sonda, so we looked it up and found it was the name of the village near the Chinese border where the Dalai Lama's mother was born.

Now, the parents have never spoken of Tibet to the child. So I said to her, "Do you know who the Dalai Lama is?" and she said, "Yes." And the parents had never spoken of the Dalai Lama either, so I said, "Who are you?" and she answered, "The Dalai Lama's mother."

So when you say fantasy, there is no fantasy. It's from a past life.

123. Several times I have run into the interesting situation of American parents having children who couldn't learn to speak English.

There was a family in New York who had twins and these children did not speak English until they were thirteen years old. They had their own special words for things and communicated between themselves. They could understand English perfectly, but just couldn't speak it.

The parents were very wealthy and brought in many linguists from around the world to try and find out what language their children were using. It was not a language that anyone knew. Suddenly, when they were thirteen they began to speak perfect English. How do you explain it?

I knew another little boy from a normal American family who had the same problem as the twins. He had his own language and could understand English, but couldn't speak it. He was having difficulty in school so they put him into a mental hospital. He was bright. He was courteous. He was polite. He was a charming youngster in every way, but he couldn't speak English.

In the hospital they tried for two years to discover what language he did speak, but they made no progress. One doctor who was watching the case was a metaphysician. He finally came to the conclusion the boy was from another planet and was born here by mistake.

124. Overindulgence of children spoils them, and then when they get out into the world they have a hard time of it. Children must have responsibility and if they don't, they grow up to be irresponsible. The whole thing in the development of any consciousness is rigid discipline. Even the meditation has to be disciplined.

For instance, a mother came to me and said her child didn't want to go to a particular school, and I said, "Does your child make these decisions?'' And she said, ''Oh yes.'' I said, ''Does your child do your banking and your business also?'' She said, ''No.'' I said, ''Of course, you do that because you are more responsible, and until he gets to the point where he can do your banking and your business, I would make these kinds of decisions for him. He must have discipline. Having no discipline is very, very bad.''

125. An adopted child is taken from an old karma to a new and better one. Many of you know D.D. His mother died when he was six months old and his father and older brother and sister took him to a family who would raise him. As they left he was held up to the window and saw them go, and he said, ''It broke my heart because I knew I had been given away.'' These children know more than we think they do.

Mission

126. You may have been given a mission many lifetimes ago and have been working towards it all this time, and now is your chance to do it. Now is the time to do it and this is why we say, do it now. Don't wait until tomorrow.

Most disciples in the Teaching are given a mission before birth. Earlier I was explaining how this far-reaching plan works. One of our disciples is slated to become Governor of New Jersey, and out in California there will be another governor, and we have people who will be in international banking, and this whole trestle board is moving together in one direction for a specific purpose.

An assigned mission is something you were born to do. This is what is meant when they speak of the ten talents. Some people invest them badly, some people throw them away, etc., but this is actually your entrusted mission; the thing you were born to do.

This is why people lose their dream and get soured on life, but if you hold onto your dream you can accomplish it no matter how impossible it may seem. It takes a dedication to what you are doing. It means to go out and create beauty for the world or bring truth; or any of these things of painting or sculpture or writing or dancing or any form of science. For instance, doctors and nurses are committed to a dream.

But how many people are doing their mission? There are thousands and thousands of people cluttering up the Earth with no justification for it. They will have to come back again and again until they catch on.

So when you realize you have a mission to do, you do it, no matter how small or how humble it may be. It may be in teaching, in medicine, in science, in any of the arts or in anything, but when you work with a dedication towards making it a better world for even one person, then you have not failed.

It was prophesied that because King Herod killed all the children at the time of Christ, he would come back as a great emperor of a country and would have a withered arm, would die in exile and be buried in a simple pine box. That was Kaiser Wilhelm, who became a woodchopper for exercise and all this came true. He was given a chance to come back and pay off his karma, but instead of doing that he made more karma.

The only difference between King Herod and Hitler, who went to Saturn, is that Herod had a mission and failed it. The only mission Hitler had was to destroy the world and he very nearly did. He was a complete dark force, and at one time it was touch and go. So, Herod had a mission and failed it. Kaiser had a mission and failed it. Napoleon had a mission and failed it; therefore, all these men are brought back until they fulfill their mission.

De Gaulle had a mission to bring France into unity, but instead of unifying France he brought disunity, so he will have to come back and undo that because he failed his mission. I had the privilege of spending an afternoon with him, and at that time he had beautiful ideals and beautiful principles. He was an idealist and had beautiful ethics, but when he came to power he became a dictator. This thing of power is very, very touchy because there is a tremendous responsibility that goes with it, and if you don't know how to handle it, you're in trouble.

Meditation

127. Prayer is talking to God or Nature and meditation is listening. In meditation you quiet the body and quiet the mind and then you are one with this flow of Nature or God. The Buddhists teach that a very good way to empty the mind is to think of a circular funnel lined with black velvet and imagine yourself in it.

If you take any question or problem that's bothering you into meditaton you will get the answer to it; maybe not the first time or the second or the third, but eventually you will get your answer. If you sit down and meditate for 15 or 20 minutes and have a good meditation, it's better than forcing yourself for an hour and getting nothing out of it. Sometimes you will have a good meditation and sometimes you will not. Sometimes you will have a magnificent one depending on how you feel and what your tensions are and how you can relax; it really is a wonderful luxury.

There are many techniques for meditation and you should use whatever works for you. I can only share with you what I have been taught and what works for me. First I still my body, and then I take a representation of God into my mind. In my shrine room I have a beautiful Buddha and I have used that image for many years. I am not a Buddhist, but Buddha means Enlightened One and I am looking for enlightenment. You can use Mohammed, Krishna, Rama; any of these great spirits. It doesn't matter. They are all representatives of God. This is your chosen image. As you cannot meditate on an abstraction—at least I can't, because mentally your mind is like a monkey in a tree—you still your body, and then you take this image and look at it until you have memorized every line and detail, and then you close your eyes and bring this up to the Third Eye and you go right out through the top of the head, just like that and you're gone. You can still the body and still the mind, but you have to have that image so you can pull it in and let go. You can do it in a streetcar, on the subway, anywhere. You direct it through the top of the head. (This is why all the monks shave their heads.)

There is another thing that will help your meditation. Hang a magnet about six inches above your head and this will stimulate the meditation.

Sitting in a lotus position puts your spine in an upright position, which is necessary for meditation. The position of the hands are up to receive. You will notice that the Buddha has one hand up and one down, meaning as above so below. We are living in both the Subtle World and the mundane world.

You may use any prayer you like, or you can make up your own prayer.

As Christ said, "Wherever two or three are gathered together in my name, there will I be also." I have often said, Christ was the greatest occultist that ever lived. Every word He ever said has great occult significance but it was lost in the translation of the Church. Anything shared is better, and that means meditation also. Meditation was cut out of the Catholic Church because they said it was worshiping idols. Not at all; they were merely used as a means of getting out of the body and that's all.

There is an exercise for opening the Third Eye: you visualize a thousand-petaled lotus and this is as white fire. You are a petal within that lotus. Now, the lotus represents God and it is solid, firm and secure. The stem goes deep down into the earth and bends neither to the right nor the left. Now bring this up to the Third Eye and hold it there for a moment and then let go. This will open your clairvoyance.

You can meditate on a symbol if you want, but know what the symbol is and what it means. The Roerich Pact and Banner of Peace symbol is very good. The three red spheres on a white background within a red circle stand for Guru, Guide and Master; or science, art and religion; or Father, Son and Holy Ghost. The red circle means immortality or life everlasting.

This reminds me of a story. This lady was very good at knitting and she was always looking for new ideas. One day she was in a Chinese restaurant and she copied some interesting looking designs from the menu which she then used on a sweater she was knitting. Later on she invited this man from China to go to dinner and she wore the sweater in his honor. He met her, and when she took off her coat, he laughed and laughed. She said, "I think you are very rude. I knitted this sweater, and I'm wearing it especially for you." He said, "I'm pleased, but do you know what it means?" "No," she said, "I copied it from a menu." Then he told her, "It means this dish is tasty and cheap." So, it's a good idea to know what you are using.

The idea of the meditation shawl is twofold. Number one, it keeps you warm. Number two, every time you meditate while wearing the shawl it builds up a vibratory rate through your aura until it becomes saturated with your vibrations. That is why if a holy man takes off his shawl and hands it to you to wear during meditation, grab it, because you will get the benefit of all his vibratory rate from it. Quite often the Swamis will notice a student who is not doing very well in meditation and they will say, "Here, take my shawl." This is a tremendous boost for them.

There was a young man who got very enthused about Vedanta. He was very devoted and a very fine person. He went to the Swami one day and said, "Swami, what about my breathing?" And the Swami said, "Pray continue."

Incense is good to use in meditation. It represents the potential in all mankind. The potential is there but, like the incense, if it is not lit, it does not function. When it is lit, it burns to ash and becomes one with infinity, and this is the potential in man, to become one with infinity.

The candle used during meditation is the symbol of fire and purity, and anything that is impure is burned by that fire. If you want to use three candles to represent the trinity, there is no reason why you can't, but there is no reason why you should. One candle, if the devotion is there, is equal to a thousand candles; however, it is not good to have the room too dark during meditation because darkness is always looking for its adversary and all adversaries of darkness are light, so you may become involved with possession.

The flower, its essence and fragrance act in a similar way to the fire by purifying and absorbing any energies that are not good.

When we say the prayer we use the gong—which later became the church bell—and every word we utter goes out on that sound and remains in infinity forever. Every word that has ever been spoken is out there in space, and one day we will have the instruments to pick up these words.

You don't need a gong or incense or flowers to meditate. If you are in the middle of the forest you cannot be carrying these things around with you. So, wherever you are, under a tree, in an old house or in a barn or by a stream, this is also part of God and this is your temple. This is just as much a temple as if it were a magnificent building, and actually you are probably closer to God.

It's wise to keep your shrines away from the eyes of the profane so as to keep them from ridicule. It's as the Mahatmas say, "We wear the white robe of immortality which we must keep spotless, not in fear of dirtying the robe, but in fear for the people who throw mud upon it, that it will spatter back upon the thrower."

Sometimes when you go into meditation you go right on into sleep. That's very good. At night when you are going to bed, lie down and meditate in bed, then let go and go right into sleep.

Don't lie down in the middle of the day to do your meditation, or lie on the floor, because that's called the corpse position; unless you are a disciple, in which case you have the protection of the Guru's aura. What may happen is an entity may enter in because you're wide open. When you're sitting up you're in full control; otherwise it's dangerous—depending on what you do and what you think and what you are, of course. During the day you also have all the vibrations and thoughts from the people in the city, and a thought can drift in very easily.

At twelve or one o'clock (A.M.) there is very little interference as most of the people are asleep. Then at two or three o'clock in the morning is when the magnetic field reaches its lowest ebb. This is when you are weakest and it's strange, but this is also when most people in hospitals die. If they live through four or five o'clock they usually live another twenty-four hours. These are the weakest hours for meditation, and between eleven and twelve at night are the strongest hours.

If you can do five minutes of being out in meditation, it's like a two-week vacation. Sometimes in meditation you may see a whole caravan pass by, or you may see city streets you've never seen before or people talking or you will see close-ups of people. It's just like a movie. Or, you may see boats or forests or complete scenes in color, with people moving.

Not long ago I was doing a meditation in which I saw a whole caravan. They all had clear skins and everyone was dressed in black with little pieces of white leather sewn all over their tunics, and I wondered where I was. It was Mongolia, and they were crossing the Gobi desert. This is an example of traveling in the astral body.

Another time, we did an experiment with one of my disciples who is a doctor. He puts people under by suggestion, not hypnosis, but by suggestion. He was very curious about the White Brotherhood and Shambhala. He knows all about this so he put me under and said, "Now I want you to go out to the Ashram of Shambhala." I was completely conscious. They had a tape and later played it back to me. I described a great wall and a gate and there was a bell. It was miserably cold. I was shivering with the cold and he said, "Ring the bell." It was a steel bell and you know I actually had a blister on my finger from touching that bell. He brought me back right away because I had no business being there.

So, this is the astral body and it can actually function in this way, but when you go out ask for protection. This is very important.

128. People often say to me, "What is the difference between sleep and meditation? I don't know if I go to sleep or if I'm meditating."

You lose all consciousness both in sleep and in meditation. The way to tell which is which is that very rarely would you sit down during the day and go to sleep during meditation if you are not accustomed to going to sleep at that time. What you do is leave the body completely. This is why in meditation you still the body and still the mind and let every part of your organism relax completely to the point of having no consciousness within you—you are gone. Only your body is sitting there.

Sometimes you may bring back scenes of experiences in meditation or you may see people or other lands or you may not. You may see absolutely nothing and not be conscious of anything. It really doesn't matter. The idea is that the meditation will relax the whole body and eliminate self. It frees your subtle body completely. If suddenly your nose is itching or your toe is hurting, you are not meditating, but you are meditating if you're completely unconscious of anything.

First, you must find a very comfortable position and it's wise to pick a time to meditate in the early morning before you go to work, say for ten or fifteen minutes, or even a five-or ten-minute meditation is better than forcing it for half an hour. Sit in a certain place every day. Be sure you are warm and comfortable. Do not try to sit in a lotus position if that's not comfortable for you.

Then just relax and you may use a personal prayer if you wish. Use any prayer you want, or make up your own prayer. Say, "I ask for help in my meditation and I am seeking spiritual wisdom and knowledge, and I ask for truth and discrimination and God Consciousness," and you've got the whole thing. As Christ said, "Ask and you shall receive." It's like the French word, *demander.* You must demand it because it's your right, your heritage and your privilege; if you don't demand it, you can stand at the door all your life and if you don't knock, it won't be opened to you.

If you establish a rhythm in your meditation, it makes it that much easier. Some people can meditate "just like that" the first time and other people take years, so it's not an easy thing. It all depends on your development.

But meditation is like a two-week vacation. You can come home after a hard day out in the babbling world, sit down and meditate for ten or fifteen minutes and feel completely rested. It lifts all of that tension. This is why it's so beneficial and this is also why they tell you in *Leaves of Morya's Garden II* to read less and meditate more. The whole secret of spiritual striving is meditation, meditation and more meditation; and then, of course, applying what you know in your daily life.

129. Whenever any group of people who are sincerely working to uplift the consciousness of mankind meet and meditate together, a little ray of light goes out into infinity, and on these rays the benevolent rays come back from the other planets. You are not just attending a class in Yoga, but you are helping these benevolent rays to come in on the rays that you are sending out. The unity of these people working for wisdom creates this ray and this is called the Cosmic Heart. If you are clairvoyant, you can see a thin stream of light emanating from these meeting places. The effect of these incoming rays are manifesting in the many changes coming about, such as whole new combinations of new ideas in education, art forms, literature, music, etc.

When you're meditating in a group and you have complete harmony, sometimes there will be a blinding flash of light accompanied by a tremendous vibration. It is just as though every part of your body is singing. It's a spirit of ecstacy that happens in a group where there is perfect harmony. That's why They speak of this over and over: harmony, harmony, harmony! It's a real experience. But if you have one person out of harmony in that room it will never work. This is why They constantly plead and stress unity and harmony. This is the only way the Maitreya can come. But you cannot send anyone away. Once the door is open, it must remain open. They can leave on their own, but that's the only way.

130. During meditation it is very good to practice exercising your imagination to the point where you experience leaving your body in astral flights. There should be no fear because nothing will happen to you. This is your birthright, your heritage and your privilege. Many times when I am traveling I get dislocated during meditation. I come back and can't find my body, but it only takes a matter of seconds to realize where I am.

There is no danger of obsession while you are out of the body. The only way you can become obsessed is if you have a very bad temper and are angry and ugly and mean to people. Only ego and anger can cause obsession.

131. A good example of discipline of the spirit is to meditate in the morning and meditate in the evening. Do your reading in the morning and at night. Many people say, "Oh, I'll skip this morning. I don't feel good or I haven't time," or the telephone rings so they say, "Oh well, I missed my time, I'll do it tomorrow." But people who make themselves do it discipline the spirit. If you make yourself do this, you will acquire what you want, but unless you do, you won't get anywhere.

132. In meditation you go out through the top of the head. When you feel your psyche going up, let go because you are sending it out. The more you do this the more you will do it automatically. It's an inner tension, but the physical body has no feeling in the arms or legs. Still your body and your mind and then your mind blanks out completely.

The whole idea in meditation is to send the astral body out. This relaxes the physical body, and all the tension is gone and all the nerves are completely relaxed. Lots of people are frightened of it, but don't be because this will add years to your life and add a great deal of youth to your body because you are getting rid of all these tensions. There is no senility when you meditate, and the mind is sharp and clear.

133. By meditating alone you can achieve a great deal, but in meditating together you each one give to the other so that your meditations should be much better because you're sharing it.

Anything shared is worth double the amount of anything not shared. Anything not shared is only for yourself.

When we would go in and meditate with the monks at the Vedanta Center in Hollywood where they had an hour meditation in the morning, an hour at noon, another hour at vespers and another hour at night, it was so terrific, you would come out at the end of an hour with a pounding headache because these men had such tremendous unity. They were there for one thing, and there was no disharmony or negativity.

Of course, you would go out and breathe in the air and your headache was gone, but the intensity was so great you could actually feel the atmosphere trembling.

After you have been there for two weeks and you go back out into Hollywood it's just as if somebody has kicked you in the stomach. I had this experience and the negative vibration that hit me was so great I was ill and had to get off the streetcar.

134. If you fall asleep during meditation, do not worry about it. In sleep you lose consciousness and between awake and asleep your clairvoyance is attuned to its highest degree. You may also be instructed during sleep and not be aware of it. You may also be performing a service during sleep and gain merit for it.

In Tibet, every Lama has between sixty and sixty-five thousand people that they work with at night. Many of these people are not conscious of this contact, or what it is that leads them into a study of these things.

In the book called *The Guru,* by Manly Palmer Hall, he tells about an English woman who did little water colors, and for thirty years she was under the influence of this Teacher and she had no knowledge of this whatsoever. Finally, the pull of India was so great she came and, of course, she met her Guru.

It was an interesting story. He wanted her to loosen up in her art. She would work very fine and tight. So he gave her this lotus and told her to study it for several days and then paint it. At the end of that time she got the whole idea that it was just the impression of the lotus that she saw and she let go. Spiritually she was also tight and by letting go in her art she could then let go and expand spiritually.

[Editor's Note: The following Meditation Prayer, Prayer of Peace, and Prayer to Shambhala have been used over the years at both the beginning and ending of meditation; therefore, it seems fitting that they should be included in the section on Meditation. The Prayer of Peace and the Prayer to Shambhala were given to my Guru by Master Morya, at the Ashram. The Meditation Prayer was most often used by Guru, with some variations.]

135. *Guru's Meditation Prayer*

We join together with our hearts
We link together with our minds
We fuse and blend our auras together
Like the colors of the rainbow
And this we offer through the heart
To our beloved Lord and blessed Hierarchy
We ask for Truth, discrimination and God Consciousness
We seek to serve and not take
May we be a light for those who have lost the way
A bridge, a boat for those who want to go to the other side
May all directions be our friend
And may we see all with the eyes of a friend
And may all see all with the eyes of a friend
May we draw closer to our Guide, our Guru and our Master
We link with the ray of the heart of the other planets
Especially Jupiter, Venus and Urusvati, Mother of the World
May our consciousness be saturated by the outer spaces
And may we be one with the entire solar system(s)
May we be filled with peace, may we be surrounded by peace
And may we give this peace to all others
We dedicate this meditation to the Ashram of Hierarchy
And to the Lord Maitreya, the coming World Teacher
To my beloved Guru, Nicholas Roerich, and to his Guru, Kuinji
Shanti, Shanti, Shanti, Aum Tat Sat, Aum Tat Sat, Aum Tat Sat
Vishnu Shakti, Vishnu Shakti, Vishnu Shakti

[Ed. Note: While the preceding Meditation Prayer was used at the beginning of meditation, the following prayer was sometimes used to end the meditation.]

Peace be unto the earth
Peace be unto the hills, the valleys, the mountains, the streams
Peace be unto all things in the air
Peace be unto all things in the sea
Peace be unto all the other planets
Peace be unto the outer spaces
Peace be unto the entire solar system(s)
Peace be unto the leaders of all countries
Peace be unto the United Nations
Peace be unto man
Peace be unto God
And Peace be unto Peace
                    Shanti, Shanti, Shanti

Prayer of Peace

136. May we, the warriors of Shambhala, unite in Love and form a ring of Light, to penetrate the prejudice of religion, and solidify to unite into Unity.

We wear the armor of the Hierarchy, that is impregnable, except by ego, anger and chauvinism. We carry our banner high over our souls, for all to see and feel.

Shanti, Shanti, Shanti

Prayer of Shambhala

137. Oh blessed Guru, Guide and Master, who guard us on the path, over barren craters, over arid deserts, over deep and dangerous ascents, through caverns deep under the mountains, through blinding blizzards and perilous passes, lead us as children. Protect us with thy shield and clothe us with the robe of immortality. Lead us to the path of labor and selflessness. Place in our hands the sword of striving and daring to smite injustice wherever it may dwell. May we be champions of the weak and oppressed. May we be aflame with love and truth. Lead us to Shambhala that we may earn the armor of the Silver Messenger. May the chalice of our hearts be filled and overflowing with love, wisdom and truth. We give our mind, we give our soul, we give our body, all and everything we are and ever will be, we surrender to God and Blessed Hierarchy. Oh Mani Padme Aum.

Karma

138. Everyone is karmically responsible for their actions whether they know about the Law of Karma or not. Any act

committed with intent by a person who doesn't know about karma is repaid tenfold. If you are a student of the esoteric and know about the law, it's one hundredfold. If you are a disciple, it's one thousandfold and if you're a Mahatma, it's ten thousandfold.

The motive is everything. For instance, if you take a life in war, your country is karmically responsible, but if there was hate in your heart when you took that life, you will be karmically attached to the family of the man you killed.

Working out your karma is a very simple thing. You say to yourself, "This is my karma, I will accept it, I will work with it, I will not object to it. I will take it and use it to learn the lesson it is trying to teach me." By doing this you will get rid of your karma, and the moment you do you will change the entire alchemy of your body.

You must remember you cannot fight karma. It can't be done. We've got to pay for it. As Buddha said, "Flow with the stream of Santana," which means flow with the stream of life, not against it, beating your head against the rocks.

When something unpleasant is happening, it's a very difficult thing to accept it and say to yourself, "Somewhere along the way I've earned this," because we always think of blaming an injustice on somebody else when all the while it is our own creation, either in this life or another one. Everything has a reason. If this were not so, life would not make any sense whatsoever. Everything would be an injustice.

But when you can say, "I must have done something to bring all this about and I am going to learn a lesson from it because all is action and reaction, as you sow so shall you reap, good for good, evil for evil, tenfold," then you can work out your karma and get rid of it.

So there is no such thing as an accident. You often hear people say, "Oh it just happened," or "This is just a coincidence." This is not true. There is always a cause and effect. I remember once when Nicholas Roerich was telling us about something that was about to happen and a man standing nearby said, "Oh, that's nothing but a coincidence," and Roerich said, "You are nothing but a coincidence."

There is good karma and there is bad karma. When you meet someone for the first time and you know them better than your own family, this is good karma. This is something very important and you should watch for it because you have been together before in a very fine relationship. Then there are the individuals you meet for the first time and for no apparent reason you dislike them intensely. They may be very charming and talented and attractive, but you can't stand to be in their presence. This is bad karma. You have had a very bad relationship with them and no matter what you do you can't get this balanced out and working.

The spirit has no relationship to the body. The parents create the body but the spirit is not of that family because it is karma to be born into any family. If a family relationship is a good one, this is good karma and you have earned that in some former life. If it's a bad family relationship, then you have been put there to learn a lesson. Many disciples are placed in such situations by their Guru to learn a particular lesson to speed up their development.

Now, in a triple karma you may have father, mother and the child that is born to them and then you have a very difficult situation. One is fighting the other and the child is fighting both. Somewhere along the line they have interfered with one another's lives.

For instance, the father may have been the son before and the child his father. The father at that time may have said, "You must study medicine," and forced him to study medicine when all his son wanted to do was be an artist or musician. This forcing of wills is not good. If you force your will, you are making karma. You are interfering with that person and you are actually playing God. The individual will harbor all that resentment and be brought back in these triangles.

If you are born into great wealth, you have earned that. If you have been born a great beauty, you have earned that also. If you are born into a family where there is culture and refinement, you have earned that. It would not be logical or right if God brought a child into the world blind or without arms or legs. This would be very unjust. This is their karma. They have done something in another life and they are paying for it. We have to pay for everything we do.

Like it says in the Bible, "Cast your bread upon the waters and it comes back tenfold." As I have said before, Christ was a great occultist, a tremendous man with this great Truth, but the Church fathers began to delete and delete. For instance, the Law of Karma was struck out of the Bible in 555 A.D. in Constantinople by the priests of the Church who boxed one another's ears and argued and fought about such pearls of wisdom as, "...do women have a soul?" and "...how many souls can you put on the head of a pin?" They also struck out the law of reincarnation, but the Bible says, "...life everlasting and immortality." What does immortality mean? Without beginning, without end. These fragments of Truth are all there but we must learn to uncover them because this is the cosmic law. The very act of striking out reincarnation and karma set back the evolution of this planet three or four thousand years. Down through the ages all the great Teachers have come to teach us these things, to bring us wisdom.

When we understand what karma is and that we have to work it out, release it and let it go, then we can eliminate it. We can't run away from it. It would be nice if we could, but we can't. If we try to run away we run right into another situation that is much worse. But if we say this is something I have created and I am going to work it out with no resentment whatsoever, then your karma is over.

You should never harbor resentment or injuries or hatreds or things of this sort because many times what may seem to be a dreadful thing that is happening to us may be a godsend in disguise. In ten or fifteen years you may look back and say, "My God, if that hadn't happened I wouldn't be here today doing this particular thing."

If everything is fine and you have no troubles or illness or anything to upset you, you have no great need for God. It's the difficulties and troubles that bring you close to the Source. But, when everything is going well and you are financially well off and have all this freedom, then you have to hang on to God with everything you've got.

139. There is a very interesting story of karma that happened some years ago when I was in Yucatan. The owner of the hotel where I stayed had been in Spain and had come home just two hours before I arrived. When I came in for dinner that night, it was very late, but he welcomed me.

Earlier in the evening I had driven in from the airport with another woman passenger. She had flown in from Los Angeles. I had come in from New Orleans. She sat in the car sobbing. I said, "Is there something I can do to help you? Are you ill?" She said, "No, no, everything is all wrong. I'm really having a nervous breakdown." I said, "Do you want to talk about it, or do you want me to be quiet or what can I do?" She said, "Well, it's a sad story." And she went on to tell me about it and as she talked she felt much better and she said, "My doctor recommended this trip, but I'm going to stay in my room and I'm not going to see the ruins. I'm just not interested." I said, "Since you've come all this distance on the doctor's recommendation, why don't you play along with him? You can't run away from your situation. I'll tell you what I'm going to do. Tomorrow morning I'm going to knock on your door and take you with us on the tour of the ruins." She said, "No, I won't go." I told her, "I promise you this, if you don't come out I'll knock your door down." She said, "I believe you would." I said, "You can be sure of it. I want to see you get rid of this nonsense you're holding onto and we'll do it by force if necessary."

The next morning she was ready to go when I knocked on her door. She wasn't too happy about it, but she went along with the tour. By the time we came in for lunch she had become so fascinated by the guide and the story of the ruins and the people that her whole attitude had completely changed.

We had lunch at separate tables because this is how it was arranged. The owner of the hotel came over to my table and said, "Mr. H., I'd like to talk to you." I said, "Surely, please sit down." He said, "I hope you won't laugh at me." I said, "I never laugh at anyone. What makes you think I would do a thing like that?"

"Well," he said, "for five hundred years my family has been Roman Catholic. I have a private chapel on my property. I go to church to please my mother and my wife, but I don't believe in the religion. I've never believed in Jesus. I have always thought He was a superstition of the Church to frighten the peons and control them." "But," he went on, "while I was planning the menu for tonight I saw the face of Christ on the right side and on the left hand side I saw your face. Now this is very significant to me. Either you are a monk or a priest or a holyman or someone like that." I said, "Well not exactly, but perhaps something like that."

That night we walked out into the fields and talked about reincarnation and healing and all of these things. He became clairvoyant and clairaudient and completely opened up. He said, "I want to take you through the ruins with this special Indian guide. I want to show you many things that are not on the regular tour." So it was arranged that we would go into the jungle for three days and see a temple that had just been discovered.

On the first night out our Indian guide said to me, "Not that I doubt you, but what is clairvoyance, clairaudience and healing? I have never heard of any of these things." He continued, "If I take you to a room in the temple can you tell me what happened there? I know what happened there, but it has never been written in a book." We went to the room. I told him, "One of the high priests was killed here with an arrow through the back of the head and it came out here and was of black material." He said, "Yes, everything you say is true. It happened right here on this spot. I have the arrow in my private museum and I'll show it to you when we get back."

Suddenly he said, "Mr. H., why does your face change? First you have a beard and now a mustache and long hair." I said, "You are seeing past incarnations." All of this opened to him just like that.

About the third day we were walking along and I said, "In there is my special home. I lived there at one time." Our guide said, "We'll cut in through the jungle." When we did, there were the ruins of a stone house. He said, "The Indians know of this house. It belonged to one of the priests who objected to the human sacrifice and they walled him up in this place and he died there."

Later we were sitting at the well where they sacrificed the virgins every year at the equinox. Two people from the hotel walked right by us and didn't see us. Amazing and terrific things happened in this part of Yucatan.

When we returned to the hotel, the owner came to me one day and said, "Mr. H., I have a problem. I have a prize bull who is very, very ill. He has an infection and I will have to kill him to save the meat, otherwise he will die and the meat will be contaminated. Is it a sacrilege to try and heal the animal?" I said, "Of course not. The bull is as close to God as you or I, maybe even closer." He said, "Could we heal it?" I said, "We can try, let's go."

It was one of those tropical storms. It was raining so hard our raincoats were soaked in minutes. We went to where the bull was lying in the mud. His sides were heaving and his heart was fluttering when he breathed.

I said, "Now, you stand right in front of the bull and I am going to treat from my heart to you and from your heart to the heart of the bull." And we began. The lightning was dancing in the sky and the thunder was rolling and the rain was coming down in buckets. In about five minutes the bull began to move and he got up on his feet for the first time in four days. He turned around and looked at me and I have never seen such a look of gratitude in all my life.

The next day the tropical storm continued and the hotel guests were all sitting on the veranda. One of the maids was running toward one of the cabanas when a bolt of lightning struck with blinding force. The next moment she was lying there and the smoke was coming out of the top of her head.

I took one look at her and I said to the hotel owner, "Grab her feet and I'll work from the top of the head." In about five minutes we hand-carried her inside. There was no brain damage, no burns, no damage to the nerves and the next day she was up and about.

It was not her karma to die. It was also probably a demonstration to the hotel owner, because I had just finished telling him that healing was his life work, that he was a natural healer, and through this incident he experienced what I meant.

140. If you find yourself in a position to help someone and you don't do it, you are incurring karma. You are there for that reason. If a man is drowning, you jump in and save him. You don't ask his age and color. If somebody asks you about the Teaching and you don't tell them but hold it to yourself, that creates karma. When you are aware of your responsibility and don't do it, that is karma.

141. In 555 A.D. when the Church threw out the Law of Karma and the Law of Reincarnation, man no longer had to be responsible for his own actions and from this point on the Church said, "For a small fee we will take care of everything. Christ died for your sins so

you don't have to worry, everything is taken care of." This is when everything went to hell in a handbasket because man *is* responsible for every action good or bad. Then the Chruch said, "We will interpret for you and we will go to God and for a small fee we will arrange all these things." But you see, no one can do that for you. You have to do it yourself. They can pray for you, but no one can forgive you your sins. If you have violated a cosmic law, you have violated it and you alone will pay for it.

There is no need for war or any of these things. If we all worked with the Law of Karma, we would know we are all brothers and sisters and responsible for one another. There would be no criminals, no divorce courts, and there would be no war. The Church has caused all the wars down through history.

It takes many lifetimes for people to realize they cannot blame others for their misfortune. But these kids know. They are catching onto this thing of karma. They know that whatever happens is their own fault and they must rectify it.

I was watching TV tonight and they were talking about the "pot" that's being smoked in the Army and why. It's because the whole thing has failed; education has failed, the Church has failed, they have all failed their mission. They have placed the full responsibility on Jesus. He died for your sins, therefore it's His fault.

All you have to do is take away the wars, take away this racial discrimination and you will have a free and beautiful people which is the normal way for people to live. If I cheat you, I am going to be cheated by ten other people, so I'm going to be darned careful how I handle each one. Those who know live that way and those who don't know live in ignorance and then say, "Why does this happen to me?"

It is a fact that Christ died on the cross, but it's a contrivance of the Church that it was for your sins. The true meaning of Christ's crucifixion was the final test of his Mahatmaship.

In a way every Mahatma is crucified. They are attacked and maligned like my Teacher was and all He did was good; like Christ and Mohammed and Buddha and Moses and all those men who have done nothing but great service, yet they have been maligned and torn to pieces because people try to pull them down to their level. When you can go through these things without hatred and resentment for what people do to you, then you have attained Mastership over self and ego and you are ready for Mahatmaship and only then. If everything is fine and rosy and beautiful and everyone is filled with love toward you, then you have no tests.

Mahatmaship is only attained on Earth because They come in from a higher planet and then They have to go through many Earthly incarnations and rub elbows with humanity in everyday life. As they say in the East, "Be in the world, but not of it," and that is the neatest trick of the week because you are not buffeted by anger or resentments or anything negative. You're free and you know that all these things are tricks of maya, of illusion, and they're false. Only the ego is affected. The ego is hurt, but what is the ego? It's nothing but a shadow.

142. In the *Letters of Helena Roerich,* there is a mistake in translation in which she says that your thought determines karma. In *The Mahatma Letters* it says, "Unless a thought is put into action it does not incur karma." If I think about giving you a beautiful painting but I don't do it, I haven't done anything. It's an empty thought and means nothing. But if I promise you a painting, then I must fulfill that promise and give it to you because I owe that debt to you, and if I don't do it in this life, then I must do it in the next and the debt then becomes tenfold.

If you do an action and it causes harm, but your motive was not to cause harm, you still have to pay the karma. Your mind should be functioning, and you should not be thoughtless and if you are, you are responsible. You are also karmically responsible for lack of discrimination.

An illustration of an exception to thought being karma was on the news broadcast from Washington tonight. The Army is condemning the officers who gave orders in the Mei Lai massacre. Now, it was their idea and while they didn't do the action, they are responsible karmically because they gave the order to destroy all those people and caused someone else to commit the action. In that case the thought was an order and the order had to be executed and all the people connected with it are karmically involved. The men who carried out the order should have known better.

Suppose you were Catholic and the Pope told you that in order to be a good Catholic you had to go out and kill every Protestant. You'd say that's insane. You wouldn't do it. It's the same thing.

In a war when you are carrying out orders against the enemy, that's a different thing, but in this case they were killing innocent people. If your country is at war and you are called to go, it is your duty to go because you are karmically connected to that country. Now, when you are faced by the enemy, you try to take them prisoner, but if you have to kill them or be killed and you don't do it in hatred you are not responsible. The country is responsible. It's the karma of your country.

If a soldier is killed, this is a sacrifice he has made for his country and his evolution is speeded up and he will come back that much faster and in better circumstances the next time. This is a cosmic law.

143. *The Secret Doctrine* and *Isis Unveiled* are great books and were dictated by the Mahatmas. HPB was maligned and ridiculed and persecuted but all this was done by the dark forces. You can always tell a dark force because they tear things down. The Teachings say, always question everything, and if you must criticize, have something better to offer in its place. One has to have discrimination.

The moment an individual condemns something and says it's vile and no good they are tearing it down to their level; therefore that person is black. I don't care whether he be a priest, minister or rabbi, when they say we are right and everybody else is wrong they are a dark force.

Criticism is fine if you have discrimination, but if you don't have a better solution to offer, your criticism is invalid. For instance, we all know that war is wrong. It's immoral and a terrible thing. That's your discrimination, but the thing is, if you protest it then you are fighting it and doing something about it. If you sit back and say it's terrible, it's horrible and do nothing about it you are still part of that karma, but the moment you protest you are free of it.

If I come to you and say something ugly about your friend and you listen to it, you are a part of that karma, but if you say, "No, I will not listen to my friend being slandered," you immediately separate yourself from it. But even by listening to it, even if you don't want to hear it or believe it you are still a part of it. It's extremely subtle but that is the way it operates. Karma is a very tricky thing.

Here is an example of how this thing works. One of my students came to me and said, "A certain person in Oxford thinks you are very cold." I said, "Oh nonsense. I may have my faults, but I don't think that's one of them." But he said, "Yes, she said this," and he named her. I said, "Ach," and threw it out of my mind, or so I thought, but do you know the next time I saw her that came right into my consciousness and it changed my whole attitude toward her and I couldn't feel the same toward her. This is how a negative thought can creep in. Finally I had to go to her and ask her about this and she said, "That's nonsense." But that's how it creeps in. It's like a worm eating and eating and you're not conscious of it. I tell you this because it's a very simple thing.

As They say in the Teaching, "We wear the armor of. . . ." But a thought is always represented by an arrow, and that arrow can put a chink in your armor and suddenly you're lost.

From now on I would just stop the individual and say, "I don't want to hear it."

144. The workings of karma can be very subtle; therefore we must be aware and observant of everything around us. If we're not,

we can miss the whole point of what it is trying to teach us. Some people will say, "Oh, that doesn't apply to me, that's for Joe Doaks over there," when they should be saying, "Wait a minute, what is this experience trying to teach me?" That's one kind of karma.

The other kind is when we say, "Okay, everything that happens to me is karma, and I accept it and don't complain and I will pay it off."

A third kind of karma is when someone is to do a special service like one of my disciples who was to go to Mars to do a special job, and since he failed that, someone else was appointed and he agreed, and so his whole karma was speeded up.

Many times people have a fixed card in *Sacred Signs and Symbols* and that means they have a fixed karma. I knew a man who came to me with this fixed karma and his wife and daughter had a fixed card, too, and the whole family had one illness after another. All their money went to pay doctor bills, but what they didn't know was that medicine would not help them; only healing by psychic energy would give them results. There are only two cards in the book *Sacred Signs and Symbols* that have a fixed karma, but when you are aware of this you can do something about it. You can always change your karma the moment you are aware of it but you have to do something about it.

Like the old German Baroness I told you about who had this nasty little apartment. It was cold in winter and hot in summer; it was small and ugly and noisy and the rent was very high. She was always complaining and I would just listen but never sympathized with her, and one day she complained that I was very unsympathetic. I said, "No, you bitch about it but you must enjoy it or you'd move." It made her so mad she went out and got a beautiful apartment at about half the rent with a garden and everything and it was warm in winter and cool in the summer. But she had to do something about it or she would be there yet. If we don't like what is happening to us we can change it.

Another example of karma is: if you are warned and told about something, be very careful to follow through on it. For example, last year a friend of mine who is an astrologer told me to be very careful between the 24th and 26th of September when going upstairs or downstairs, as I could fall and have a very bad accident. She said, "I've gone over your horoscope and this is the indication, and a word to the wise is sufficient." So for those two days whenever I went up or down the stairs I held onto the handrail. On the 26th I caught my heel in the rug and I fell forward, but my hand was on the rail so I caught myself and got my balance. This was at the top of the stairs and had I not been holding onto the railing I would have fallen all the way down the stairs and had a very bad accident. But this is the way you head off karma because I was willing to listen.

That's how psychic energy works to warn the individual and this is an extra protection. This is another reason why you are given this energy so that you can use it to protect people, if they are willing to listen. Of course if they aren't willing to listen that's their karma too.

We may know all the laws of karma and all about psychic energy and have all the experience of a great yogi, but if we don't do something with this and put it into action it's of no value.

Most karma is action, but sometimes we have the karma of inaction. This means we should not interfere with another's karma. For instance, if you want to study architecture and your mother says, "No, you can't, you must study law," she is interfering with your development and that's karma.

Someone asked me about failing to do something that we know is right. If you don't do it, there is not punishment for that. You must remember that everyone has absolute free will. Now if you have an idea and you don't do anything with it, somebody else will take that idea and do it. Like the man who was sitting meditating and another man came along and said, "What are you doing sitting there under that tree doing nothing?" He said, "I'm building a temple." "Where are you building it?" "In the Subtle World." Somewhere on the other side of the Earth an architect is picking this up and is designing a temple on his drawing board. He goes out and buys wood and glass and steel and he is building this temple, so what looks like an inaction may be a terrific action.

Like the story of the two glasses of water, one with salt and one without. What you see you cannot believe unless you taste it, but even if you can't see it, it's there.

145. When you know that karma is the basis and cause of everything, then you have the key to life. You will have no resentment, no anger and you can say, "This is my karma, I've earned it. If it's good, I've earned that and if it's unpleasant I've earned that too, either in this life or the last."

A friend of mine, a German Baron, kept going to the slums on the lower east side of New York and he would tell me, "This upsets me. It tears me to pieces. I would like to do something for these people." I said, "This is their karma. They were probably very wealthy at one time and let people starve. Their karma has placed them there so they can learn. I feel sorry for them because they are ignorant, but if they hadn't made mistakes they wouldn't be in that position." If you are born to great wealth you have earned it and if you are born to great poverty you have earned that too through your past lives, but what you do with your life is another thing.

For instance, Billy Rose was born in the tenements on the Lower East Side of Jewish parents. He was a little man, about five feet tall, frail and delicate and very poor. He became a millionaire and left one of the greatest art collections in New York City. Did he stay in the gutter and cry? No, he did something about it.

So don't sit down and give up but keep striving and you will get there in spite of yourself, but you have to have that drive to do it. If you want to become a great artist, or a millionaire, or a great mathematician, or a general, or a mechanical genius, you can. These things are all within you. They are only sleeping. Wake them up, utilize them.

It's true, these people on the East Side may not have an education, but there are free night schools. They'd rather drink beer and watch television and let someone else so their thinking for them.

As Buddha said, "Men cry and complain when all around them is light and illumination beyond the wildest dreams of man, and all you need do is reach out and touch it."

146. Many times disciples are placed in a family for a definite reason. No, they are not always told. This they must find out for themselves. As in the East, you have to continuously ask, "Who am I and why am I here?" You may have developed one talent and be working toward one purpose, but the Teachings say we must be able to do three things that are creative to be a well-rounded individual, and everything is creative. You can make office work creative. You can make washing dishes creative. You can make digging ditches creative. You see, it's what you put into it.

A long time ago I talked to a lady who was very, very lazy. She was having a lot of problems that had gone on for many, many years. She came to me and said, "I would like to ask your advice." I said, "Okay." She said, "I'm having all these problems and I don't know why. I know there is such a thing as karma, but I don't understand why all this is happening." I said, "Well, do you want me to tell you the truth? It's going to be kind of a shocker." She said, "Yes, I do." I told her, "Your problem is you are lazy. Now if you can accept that and work it out, fine, but if not, that obstacle is going to stare you in the face until you get rid of it."

The interesting thing was that she took two jobs. She said, "If I'm going to break out of this, I'm going to have to do it with not one job but two. I've got to make up for the time I've been sitting around doing nothing." She ended up owning the restaurant that she started working in on a part time basis. She said, "It's the most wonderful life as long as you keep moving." This is true, but the moment we sit down and stop this means we're satisfied with what we have and there we sit.

So this is overcoming karma, and you too can overcome your karma. Instead of doing just so much on your job, always do more than is expected of you. When you see somebody is in trouble, go to them and say, "Can I help you?" and in this way you are creating harmony in the world. Many times you've heard it said, "People will take advantage of me." No one can take advantage of you because you are giving. Now, this is the trick of karma. The more you give the more you receive. This is why people cut themselves off when they will not give. Usually it's because they are afraid. As Christ said, "Ask and you shall receive. Knock and the door shall be opened to you." Instead of going 50/50, go 70/30 and you will be building a very good karma.

This is true in everything. If you go to school and bring to the teacher respect and love and devotion, you will get from that teacher what he himself does not have because your attitude is right and with that attitude you gain and not the teacher. This is also true of employers. Go back to President Kennedy's words, "Ask not what your country can do for you but what can I do for my country." This is a great occult esoteric secret of karma, but it's not for lazy people.

147. The expression, "Only the good die young," means they don't have to go through life with all its bitterness and disillusionment. Their karma for that life is ended.

Actually, we are taught the wrong concept of death. We are taught when you're dead you're dead and that's all there is to it, but death is no more than walking through that door and coming in another door with a new body; but the consciousness always remains. We have been dead hundreds and hundreds of times, so when you can get rid of this fear of death then you are free of all the hang-ups of karma. That's why in the West they hate the word karma and fight like hell against it. They associate it with dying and coming back over and over again, but we only come back to learn lessons.

Earth is a great schoolhouse. As Shakespeare said, "All the world's a stage...play your role well," which means, "Why am I here? What is my purpose? How best can I serve humanity?" When you know what that role is, you need not come back unless you want to serve and then you ask, "Where can I best serve?" It may be Mars, it may be here. The need is very great, for wisdom is a rare thing and learning the whole thing of karma is actually learning the wisdom of life.

148. We had a case in New York of a young lad who was dead for three minutes and was brought back to life with no brain damage. This is miraculous. It is an interesting story of karma involving a man and his son. This young man had a tremendous healing. He was healed

of epilepsy and told never to drink or smoke again, ever, or he would have more epileptic fits. Occasionally, however, he would take a drink.

One night he had an argument with a couple of men who were drunk. He shouted at them and they began to beat him. They threw him against the steering wheel of his car and he hit the wheel with his neck. There was no mark but the entire windpipe area began to swell. It choked off his oxygen supply and he turned blue. He was taken to the hospital where the doctors made an opening in his windpipe and inserted a tube so he could breathe.

He was coming along very well and was out of the hospital. On Sunday his father called me and said, "I have a feeling that something is going wrong with my son. Can you tell me anything?"

I said, "I don't know what it is but be ready to have him and his doctor at the hospital on Wednesday at four o'clock because something important is going to happen one way or the other. He may suddenly get well or he may die. It's touch and go and it's four o'clock on Wednesday."

This man is one of the few people who, when he asks for advice, will follow it straight through right to the letter. He called the doctor and at four o'clock he and the boy were at the hospital.

Suddenly the boy stopped breathing and he was dead for three minutes. They opened him up and massaged his heart and brought him back to life. If the doctor had been two or three minutes late the boy would have died.

I was so impressed by this incident because the boy is an impossible teenager. He is in trouble all the time. I have no idea why he was saved. Evidently he has a special job to do in this life or the Hierarchy wouldn't have gone to all the trouble to give a warning including the exact day and hour.

We got a very interesting reading on this boy. He was a Nazi German flier in the last World War (WWII) and he has come back. He loves the German language. He studies it and speaks it like a native. He collects swastikas and loves planes and guns and knives. Only Hierarchy knows why he was saved.

There is another story about this boy's father. He was in the British Air Corps in Africa during World War II. One day he was left in charge of the barracks. He got so sleepy that he lay down on a cot and went to sleep. He says that he sleeps like the dead. Normally you can shout and holler and yell; nothing will wake him.

But on this particular day he heard his name called in a normal tone of voice. He jumped up and ran out of the building just as the whole place blew up behind him. It had been hit by a shell. He was saved because someone had spoken his name and it woke him.

Evidently, both he and his wife and son have had the shield of protection of Hierarchy all their lives.

149. Another illustration of how this karma works, absolutely perfectly: this young man brought his young lady over to introduce her to the Teaching. She was a very lovely girl, an artist and dancer. We spent the evening talking about the Teaching. They left and as they were crossing the street a car came along and hit her. The boy said it felt just as if someone had grabbed him by the trousers and pulled him back, but she was hurt. Her leg was broken.

He ran back to get me. He came running in and said, "They hit her! They hit her!" I ran to the bedroom and got a blanket and pillow because I knew she would be in shock. By the time we got to the street the police had already arrived. Normally they will never let you touch anyone who has just been injured. One of the officers, who must have been very new, went to pieces. So his partner came over and asked me to help him.

I said, "Of course." We put the girl on the stretcher; then he said, "Will you help me get her into the ambulance?" I did. "Will you ride with her to the hospital?" I did and was able to treat her all the way and relieve her pain.

This is how karma works. The impossible happens. Ordinarily the police will never allow you to help them at the scene of an accident.

Now you will ask, "Why did the accident happen?" She was a nice girl with a very good mind, but she was very poor and had never traveled. She had never gone anywhere. Because she was hurt in an accident, she received a settlement from the insurance company that allowed her to travel all over Europe for three years. This changed her whole consciousness, her whole life.

That which was bad turned out to be very good. Many times an obstacle that looks like something very bad turns out to be a blessing in disguise. We all know that by the tragedies that have happened to us we have grown. We've all gained and benefited by our difficulties.

150. Is there an energy that compels you to fulfill your karma? Yes, if you feel a great need to do something, you may as well go ahead and do it. It's going to come out somehow and it may as well be now as later. We're talking about sensible things, not foolish or stupid things.

For example, there was a man and woman in Canada who were very wealthy. The husband was one of those men who came up from the bottom. He had very little background, but was a fine and wonderful person.

His wife came to me and complained that he wanted dinner

parties every night. He wanted the biggest car and the best, the biggest, the most expensive of everything. They had to have more servants than anyone else in town and more of everything. She said, "I'm going crazy. I love my husband; he is a wonderful man, but this is awful. We are never alone. It's like living in a hotel. We're never together and he continues to want all this extravagance."

I said, "These things are not important to you because you are accustomed to wealth. You've had all the money you wanted. You've traveled all over the world. Your husband never had any of this. He has never had these experiences before. He needs them and wants them so give it to him. Instead of having ten people for dinner, have twenty. Instead of going to bed at one o'clock, make him stay up until three. Give him plenty of excitement until he hollers 'Uncle'! Then, you can taper off and live a happy life." That is exactly what she did and it worked. He had to go through that experience to learn from it.

151. Many people have the idea that to have a lot of money is evil. It isn't. It's what you do with it and your responsibility for it that's important. If you have a great deal of money, you have earned that right and you also have a great deal of responsibility to use it wisely. If you don't, it will be taken away from you. You might come back next time as a very poor individual and die of poverty. So there again everything that happens is karma. If we can accept that we have the whole answer to life.

152. The question is often asked: "How do you make a value judgment between helping people and interfering with their karma?"

If the individual asks for help, you immediately help them. You can offer to help but if they don't want it then don't push it on them, because that's violating their karma. For instance, if an individual doesn't want a healing, you walk off and leave them. You can pray for them that whatever can happen that is good for them will happen, but you can't pray for them to get well. If you pray for them to get well and they do, you're forcing your will on them. If someone is in pain you can pray that their pain be eased, but you can't pray it be taken away unless they ask you, because with the will you can change anything, no matter what it is.

153. It's an old Christian idea that God is punishing us. This is nonsense. We are not being punished for anything. We are paying for the things we did in our past life or in this one.

If you want to you can eliminate all your karma in one lifetime. The Mahatmas are like a cheering section. They will cheer you on but they are not going to tell you how to play the game. You have to work that out for yourself. If you are having a beautiful life, you know you have earned that, and if you are having a dreadful time, you know you have done something wrong.

When you have worked out all your karma and you have fulfilled your mission on Earth, then you become a Mahatma and you can create your body at will. The whole idea of the Mahatmas is to help and to serve, but they will not do your work for you. They will indicate and make suggestions but you have to follow through on it.

154. Earlier this evening we were talking about karma and Napoleon. He didn't follow orders so he will have to come back and work this out. Josephine was his contact with the Hierarchy. Through her he was instructed on every battle and every movement in France, and he followed through except for one thing. He was told, "Never declare war on Holy Russia," but he wouldn't listen, and he did and so lost it all.

His job was to build France back into a very powerful nation, which he did, but because he threw it all away he has to come back again and fulfill this mission and bring France back to a very high level of spiritual consciousness, culture and art.

There is a prophesy that any day now (1971) you will see a young man about 38-40, a young captain, who will become Premier and will be Napoleon and will restore France back to her original position. So this is a karmic debt he has to pay.

155. This country has incurred very bad karma for the bombing of Hiroshima and Nagasaki, and we are incurring even more in this Viet Nam War because it is illegal, immoral and wrong.

It's true the bombs were the only thing that stopped the war or it may have gone on for a long time, but an action like that is a great responsibility and it is the country's karma, and we are part of that karma whether we approve of it or not.

It's like the Viet Nam War, we are against it and we protest and work for peace, but we are part of that karma because the United States is our country and we are part of that country.

156. If you meet a Jew from England or Germany and you ask him, "Who are you?" he will tell you, "I am English or German." But if you ask a Jew in America, "Who are you?" he will tell you, "I am Jewish."

This ties the person to the karma of that particular group, instead of first assimilating the country they live in and then saying, I am of the Jewish religion.

I was talking to a man today and he asked me, "What is your religion?" I said, "I am a Christian, a Mohammedan, a Buddhist, a Jew, every religion in the world." He said, "I don't understand you."

The same thing happens to the man who is colored. When he says, "I am a Negro," he separates himself immediately. I have a very dear Negro friend, a wonderful old man, and he said, "It took me thirty-five years to get over being a Negro. I decided one day to be everybody's brother and then I discovered there was no difference between us. The difference was that big chip on my shoulder and there were a lot of people ready to knock it off."

157. Being born is karma and you begin paying it off from the moment of birth. You may be born into a wonderful family and have a wonderful relationship or you may be born into great wealth and position. You have earned that. People who have great beauty have earned that because their souls and consciousness have been beautiful, and so they bring this in with them. Of course, what they do with it is another thing. People born to great poverty have earned that. In another life they may have abused all sorts of privileges, so this time everything is taken away and they must learn their lesson.

We are all sum and substance of everything we have ever been in all our past lives. What we are is not the result of just this one life. As I have said before, you know how to grow your own body but you have forgotten how to do it. Your father and mother supplied the body and fed it but you grew it. All your essence, everything, is in the subconscious area of your being. You have to tap this and pull it out and this is called metaphysics, or beyond physics. All men and women have these great possibilities within them, but they don't use them. The idea is to bring out all the qualities and talents that you have, so you can work as a total person. If we can make this a better world for even one person, it justifies our existence for cluttering up the Earth.

We may go to school and study for years, but wisdom comes from living with people, working out problems, working out prejudices and hatreds and all of these things until we can live in peace and harmony with all the wisdom we can bring forth. When you can throw off all this pettiness against creed, color and religion, etc., then you're working toward Mahatmaship.

158. We are never born into a situation we can't handle. For instance, I met an engineer in Cedar Rapids, Iowa who has only one finger and one thumb. He was born that way. He's a draftsman and a very good one. He works by placing the pen between his teeth. He makes eight or nine dollars an hour (1967) because he's that good. He has a great handicap but he doesn't allow it to stop him.

159. Sacred karma is when a student or probationary does a great service for the Hierarchy. Good karma is earned. An example of this are the five teachers connected with the New Age School in

Texas who all got their initiations, and in California a couple who had been on probation for ten years opened a New Age School and got initiation for that act.

The fastest way to God Consciousness is through selflessness and sacrifice. For instance, the kings and queens are little understood. They are born into that karma to help their country. They have no life of their own. They have no love life of their own. They cannot marry whom they choose. This is their duty because this is the position they were born into and if they follow through, this is their higher karma and the gates of karma are open to them, but if they don't follow through they may come back as a beggar. "Many a king walks the Earth in beggar's rags for things done and left undone."

Another example are the Kennedys who were all millionaires and could have been playboys, but they sacrificed their lives, and for this they earned sacred karma.

160. One of my disciples kept complaining, "Why didn't I get this Teaching until I was fifty?" I said, "I don't know, dear, it must have been your karma." One day we were having breakfast at the Ashram and she said, "I just remembered something. When I was sixteen years old I was invited to the Roerich Museum and I could have met Nicholas Roerich." I said, "There's your answer. Why didn't you go?" She said, "I would never do what I was told." So it took a few years. Oftentimes being bullheaded is very costly, but as They say, if we miss the boat once we'll be given another chance in seven years.

161. There is an old saying, "Never leave a bed unmade." This is true. As I've said many times, if you leave an apartment or house for the next tenant, never leave it sloppy or dirty. If you do, you're going to move into a place ten times dirtier. You are preparing it for the next person. Karmically you owe that.

162. The karmic husk—I can best explain this by giving you an example. This young lady had been engaged to a man for eighteen years, and it had been a constant battle back and forth. She came to me and asked why they couldn't get together. I said, "I'd rather you ask yourself that question and when you have the answer come and tell me. If I tell you, you will accept it on intellectual grounds and you may feel that maybe it's right and maybe it isn't, but like all esoteric things, if you put it to the test, then it's an experience and you know firsthand, not secondhand."

She came to me about six months later and said, "Now I know why." And she told me this story. In a former life in Italy, she was Jewish and he was a Roman. Now he is Jewish and she is Catholic, and he has a very bad inferiority complex about being Jewish.

In this former life the Jews were confined to a ghetto. The gates would be opened at sunrise and closed at sunset, and during this time the Romans would often ride through the streets. So she met this man who was Roman and they fell in love. At this time there was a very strict law that said if a Roman married into another religion, their wealth would be taken away from them. So he would come to the ghetto every day and eventually they had a child.

He spoke to his mother who was a very wise woman and she said, "We will give out that this is the child of a relative. The mother died and we are bringing this woman to be its nurse. In this way she can bring up her child and the servants will know her as a nurse, and you can live together secretly."

A few years later the father was killed in a chariot race. The boy and his mother stayed on, and when he was about sixteen the grandmother died and on her deathbed she called the grandson in and said, "This is not your nurse. This is your mother." The boy became very angry and threw the mother out and sent her back to the ghetto.

One night he was riding in the ghetto and she was walking across the square and his horse knocked her down and as she lay there realizing her back was broken, she looked up and recognized the face of the man she was involved with in this life. It was her son who had killed her. The whole thing flashed across her memory.

This was their karmic husk. Had they married it would never have worked out, because they were too karmically entangled. It could only be resolved when they realized what had happened and then doing something intelligent about it. Instead of trying to force a marriage, they need to say, here it is, we are involved in this, and then release it.

The interesting thing of karma is that we have earned whatever happens to us, either in this life or in another or another. If we can get rid of this karma, we break these relationships and we won't have these ugly things happen to us.

This is the whole idea of Milton's *Paradise Lost*. This is a paradise, but it's the karma we have made that keeps us from realizing it.

In all Christian religions, they say, "Cast thy bread upon the waters and it will come back tenfold." This is the tenfold law of karma. If I do something good for you, tenfold good will come back to me, not from you, but from ten other sources. If I do something evil, I'm going to have to pay for that tenfold also. Many people have a hard time in life because of not knowing about the Law of Karma which was struck out of the Christian religion in 555 A.D. in

Constantinople by the Catholic Church. This is the law of cause and effect. That's what karma is.

Christ was a great occultist. He taught, "Vengeance is mine saith the Lord." You don't get even with anyone. You leave that up to karma. It will repay better than you ever could.

In the East they say if you help another person, you help yourself more. And if you keep it a secret, you receive tenfold in return.

Lords of Karma

163. The Akashic records are like a great filing system. Everything you have ever been or thought or done from the beginning of your existence, even if your source of origin was from another planet, is recorded there. Everyone in the world has such a record. As Christ said, "As a man thinketh so is he," and this too is part of the Akashic record.

No one has access to the complete Akashic record except the Lords of Karma, not even the Dhyan Chohan. There are times when your stars may be in conjunction with those of a clairvoyant person for a period of a few minutes to an hour or so, and then they may have access to certain developments in your record, but never the whole thing. So when people say they can read your entire Akashic record, don't believe them. No one has that right, except the Lords of Karma, because sometimes they need to change your karma. They can do that and it does happen. Actually this is what karma is; you pay off the debts in these Akashic records.

164. The question is, "What is a cosmic vortex?" This is the whole Law of Karma from other lifetimes. Then there are the Akashic records and, as I said earlier, you are responsible for every action in those records. Now this is a vortex and you can tune in on that vortex.

As we were talking earlier, if you suddenly feel a great peace come over you, this is part of that vortex and your connection with it allows you to feel this. All absent treatment in healing is part of this vortex. And when you are sensitive and aware, you are also utilizing this cosmic vortex.

When they speak of the spiral, this is the ascension of the consciousness of your quality and the more you ascend the more you are able to tap that vortex any time you want and use it as a power.

165. Free will is very important. For instance, a Mahatma may appear to you and say, "I want you to do a certain mission, if you wish." It's never imposed on you. And you say, all right I'll do it, but then you say I've got a play coming up and I can't do it now, I'll do it later. The mission is given to someone else.

Karmically, the person to whom the mission is now given may be nearing the end of their life cycle, but the Mahatmas will come and say, "Do you mind hanging around twenty or thirty years longer because this chap has dropped the ball and failed to do this, so if you will take on this mission we will make this extension." And they actually change your karma. Now you don't have to do it and they don't threaten you; it's only if you want to do it because this thing of free will is terribly important.

That actually happened to me because of someone in California who failed a mission. I knew exactly when I was to be killed in a plane accident. I already had my ticket, but They told me to cancel the flight if I would do this mission instead. So here I am. That was around 1947, 1948. The plane I was to have taken did crash on the mountain top.

All the disciples who have come in after this have had their karma speeded up because I would have taken them in the next life. It meant changing the karma of every one of these people, but the Lords of Karma have access to the Akashic records and can do this.

There is no guess work. When you are ready, the Teacher appears. I was given the name and picture of each disciple sometimes twenty years before. As Christ said, "Many are called but few are chosen." It all depends on what you do with striving and devotion and working. As Jesus said, "The first shall be last and the last shall be first." The last person you would expect may sometimes be first and the one who has all the qualifications may sometimes be the last.

Another example of how the Lords of Karma operate is this great and wonderful thing that happened with B., who has been with me now seven years. He's a teacher of chemistry and English in New York (City).

About the second week he was with me he heard me make the statement, "You must never ask the teacher if he is your teacher, because if you don't know and are not sure, then the answer has to be no. It's halfwayness and you must know completely." So, immediately he said, "Are you my teacher?" I said, "I just got through telling you the answer. The answer is no." Evidently he was doing this to show me he didn't give a damn.

Now in the seven years he's been working with me, he's cried about this thing and I said, "Look, B., I'll do everything I can to help you find another teacher. This I promise you, because I like your work and I like what you do, and I know you are sincere and I know when you asked that question you had been three years in analysis and were all mixed up, but what has been said has been said and I can't change that, or take it back. If it were up to me I would take it back, but it's not up to me. I can't do it."

So at Christmas he was here (at the Ashram) and he said, "I know that someone failed on their mission to Mars." We are a group going to Mars to do special work. He said, "If I offered myself to the Hierarchy to go to Mars, would they accept me?" and I said, "Surely." He said, "Well, I offer myself completely. Let them do with me what they will."

When I went into New York the following week he said, "Look R., if I were your disciple I could serve you better," and I said, "This is true, but I have no control over what has happened. This is cosmic law and karma and I cannot change it. I have no right whatsoever." He said, "Would you ask your Guru or the Lords of Karma if they would make an exception in this case so that I can be of better service?" I said, "Well, I'll ask." So I wrote the letter and burned it. This is the way it's done; but nothing happened for about a week and a half and when I was on my trip to the West Coast, I got the answer, yes, yes, yes.

So the Lords of Karma evidently worked on this, and because he was willing to sacrifice himself for this mission They said yes. I told him, "Now I can take you on probation," but that's the first time that's ever happened. I tell you this to show you how the Lords of Karma operate. There is always an exception to the rule no matter how hard the rule is, depending on the sincerity of the person and their devotion and their dedication.

This is like a great game of chess and we are the chessmen, and we are moved about and the Lords of Karma and the Dhyan Chohans are all watching this play over our shoulders. Agni Yoga was meant for everyone but so few have come. I quote from the Teaching, ". . . do not count in hundreds or thousands, it exists in tens." It is not quantity but quality that counts, for whenever there are diversified people working together with heart and love we are ten thousandfold strong. So you don't need great crowds of people. When I travel around to the various groups, everywhere there is this terrific unity, this wonderful quality of love and you can actually reach out and touch it.

166. Years ago there was a young flier who came to us who was very interested in Vedanta. He was a very pure soul and had this very

close, beautiful relationship with M. so that M. would give him instructions through me and would tell him what to watch for and what to do, etc. One time he came to me and said, "Do the boys upstairs have any instructions for me?" And I said, "Yes, you are going down to the Bahamas (he was a flier for Pan Am), and when you land watch over the landing gear. You must not say a word. You will have a slight crash but no one will be hurt. You will be shown a safety device so that this accident will never occur again. You must not cry out or say anything or you won't see it."

Later he was telling me that when they came in for a landing the pilot put down the wheels but only half way down and then he forgot and they landed on their belly and broke the propellers. He said, "As this happened, I looked and there on the panel was a red light that went on and off. It had never been there before." Now, every plane has a flashing red light to tell them when the landing gear is down. Before this they had no way of telling.

For the next several flights there were no instructions. Then he was flying to Africa and he asked, as always, but M. said, "No, nothing going over, everything will be routine, but on the way back you must look at the first gas tank on your left side. The nuts have fallen off from the vibration and are in the tank, and the motor is resting on just these bolts. When you get over the ocean the vibration will shake the whole wing off and the plane will go down."

He said, "Okay." So they flew over and everything was routine. He went into town and when he came back they had the plane all gassed up. The tank on this wing had about 400 gallons of gas in it. So he said, "Drain it." They protested and complained but he persisted and when they got the gas out the motor was resting on the bolts, and the nuts were on the gas tank.

By following instructions he saved the lives of the passengers and crew. I tell you this story to show you how karma can be changed, otherwise that whole group of eighty-six people would have been lost.

167. As a rule a murdered man must live out his normal life span on the astral plane. If it was an act of karma he can come back right away, but if it was an act of carelessness he must spend the rest of his days waiting in the Subtle World until his life span is up and only then can he come back. But the murdered one, depending on whether he has very important work to do, may come back very quickly.

If it's a murder of violence or hatred he has to live out his life span, and usually when these people come back they have a karmic tie. To illustrate this, when Ghandi was falling and a split second before he died he said, "Forgive this man and remove his karma for this act." Instead of thinking, "I've been shot, I'm going to die," his first thought was to plead for the release of this man from his karma. Now, whether he would be released or not is a question for the Lords of Karma. Usually whatever we are working out here is karma from this life or another one or several others.

War

168. The New Age began in 1936. Armageddon began on the subtle plane in '36 and in the mundane from about 1945 on.

The war in Viet Nam is very bad, but the prediction is that it will bring about the end of all wars. People will get so fed up and so sick of it they will do something about it, and when people will live in peace among themselves and practice peace we will have peace on Earth, but it is going to come from the people themselves and from their consciousness. As we change the world will change, and by our example we can be a tremendous influence. As Roerich always said, "Be an example to others." You don't have to talk about the Teaching, you don't have to shout, you don't have to tell anything, just be.

This change in the consciousness of people will take place gradually because of the conditioning of their minds over the centuries. For instance, our churches have accepted war, and the people have accepted war as their duty, and they will have to change that whole conditioning of their minds before peace can come. We are not English, or French, or German, or American. We are people of one planet, therefore we have to learn to live in peace. If we can't do that, how in the world can we talk about brotherhood. Brotherhood has no chauvinism.

In the same way we have been conditioned by taxes. I can remember when there were no taxes on the phone, no taxes for traveling, no taxes for the theater. These were all imposed during the Second World War. Gasoline taxes, for example, were imposed to prevent people from traveling unnecessarily, but people have continued to pay these taxes because they're used to it, they're conditioned.

This conditioning is in the schools, in the colleges. It's a terrible thing when individual thinking has been thrown out. It's mass thinking and you must think this way or you're a dirty communist. If you disagree with the group in power, you're an activist and that's a dirty something else. They tell you in the Teachings you have to fight constantly for your individuality.

The newspapers are either Republican or Democrat and each one slants the news to its own way of thinking, to suit the owner of that paper. The only paper that is free of any bias is the Christian Science Monitor and it gives very little news of world events.

This conditioning is something we have to fight constantly.

169. "What about going to war?" is one of the questions that is often asked. I tell many of my students, "You have a karmic link with your country and it's wise to go through with it because you will have that protection anyway and you will also discharge that karma, whereas if you run away because you're frightened your protection is not there."

An illustration of this happened to one of my disciples when he was a student at the university in Cuba. There were a group of students who were plotting to overthrow Batista, and three of them were elected to go to this particular place and steal some ammunition. It was a very dangerous mission in which they might all be killed.

The leader of the group sent himself a wire saying he had to go to the other end of the island because his mother was dying. So he went home to his mother who lived opposite a club. In the evening he walked across the street to this club and he heard an argument going on inside and he looked in the window and someone pulled a gun and shot him. So he ran away from death only to find it.

Now, my disciple and the other man went to the guard of the ammo dump and he said, "You can have all the ammunition you want. Just tie me up so it looks good and you can have the whole thing and welcome to it." You see, they were protected and there wasn't a shot fired.

In war, if you have to kill, this is the karma of your country as long as you do it without hate for the enemy. And if you are killed you will come back into a better environment. This thing of war is a very tricky thing of karma because there is personal karma, national karma, and world karma and any injustice must be fought wherever it may dwell, and if we stand by and do not protest we become a part of it.

170. There was a gunner in World War II whose plane was hit by the Germans. He was knocked out and had no parachute. He fell something like three or four thousand feet. The next thing he knew he was lying in a field. He felt himself and found no broken bones. Ordinarily he would have been about eight feet underground.

He got up, tore off his uniform and, disguising himself as a road worker, walked down the autobahn painting a white line down the middle of the road with a paint brush. This is how he got out of Germany and rejoined his unit.

The men in his squadron had seen him fall and they knew he had no parachute. When he rejoined them it was as if he had returned from the dead. They thought he was a ghost.

I told this story in San Jose, California and a man came up to me afterwards and said, "I was the pilot of that plane and I knew that gunner very well. I can authenticate the story."

I read of a child who fell out of a six-story window onto the pavement and there wasn't a broken bone or bruise.

These things happen because of karma, and also because it is not their time to go.

Prophesies

171. There are warehouses full of unfulfilled prophesies and predictions because of changes in karma. Recently I read that the Duchess of Windsor is going to have the title, Your Royal Highness, restored to her. When this happens it will change the whole karma of the Windsor family. It doesn't seem like much on the surface and not terribly important, but their stuffy old attitudes are going and they are undoing a wrong by doing the right thing. When we undo a wrong we right that karma, and then the whole karma is settled.

We have karma of country, karma of family, karma of religion, karma of color, karma of creeds, karma of philosophy; so you see everything is karma, everything that we associate ourselves with.

172. The prophesy is that there will be a shifting of poles and as a consequence there will be erratic changes in the weather, especially in the southern states. There will be whole land mass shifts. One of the shiftings occurred in India and Pakistan—where there were so many people lost recently. This is the prophesy. Japan will sink overnight. There will be a few mountains left but the rest will go under.

Karmically, it is the time for the people caught in these catastrophies to go. When you consider that all is karma, if it isn't meant for some people to go, they won't. They will be away or visiting. For instance, when Long Island goes, the people who are working in some sort of Teaching will be sent away or told to go or be pulled away for a purpose.

Long Island is sitting on an ice ledge. The gulf stream is shifting and this will melt the ice underneath. Already the tropical fish from the gulf stream are being washed up on the beaches. New York itself is on a solid rock so nothing will happen to it.

I have a map marking all the volcanos, active and inactive, in the world and you would be amazed at how many there are. The inactive ones can become active because they are all linked underneath. It's like a ring of fire. For instance, San Francisco is sitting on two volcanos. One is about five miles out and the other one is Nob Hill. The Millionaire Club is built right on top of it. Besides San Francisco, Bakersfield and Vancouver all have volcanos, and then the ring of fire goes out into the ocean to the Aleutian Islands and Japan and Java and the tip of Peru and there is a complete circle. Then there is a ring of fire on the other continents. There is a prediction that Moscow will be a seaport and that Greece will be nothing but a series of islands and the Rock of Gibraltar will be no more.

173. One of the things that the Mahatmas tell you is that the mass mind is not intelligent. If you are going to work with something, you must be thoroughly informed and have the intelligence to know what you are doing. The mass mind is not informed and they do stupid things.

You must have leaders who are good, who are intelligent, who are spiritual, who are thinkers and then they can lead the masses. This is what happened in France at the time of Louis XVI. The best brains were killed off and this is why France is suffering today.

There is a legend that Napoleon, who was sent by the Hierarchy to do a special work—and which he did up to a certain point—was told never to invade Holy Russia or his reign would end in catastrophe. All invasions of Russia have ended in catastrophe, because basically they are working with the Orthodox Russian and Greek philosophy which is completely esoteric and occult. This is why it is called Holy Russia. Many of their priests are clairvoyant and clairaudient and are healers, so they operate on a very high spiritual principle.

The prophesy is that out of the present-day Russia will come the school of the Bodhisattvas. This will be one of the great living schools like the schools of Plato and Socrates and will blossom again with great wisdom and knowledge. These schools will also be found in Alexandria and Cairo; in County Cork, Ireland; in Istanbul, Turkey and in the heart of Greece.

The book, *Psychic Discoveries Behind the Iron Curtain,* is the handwriting on the wall. This is happening through science and not through the Church; and by reaching out into another dimension and acquiring it in this way, the rest of the world will accept it because it is pure science.

Reincarnation

174. Krishna is a craving for life and according to his karma man will be brought back into life. It's man's desires that bring him back over and over again.

Take for instance a man who is greedy for money, a miser. This karma will hold him to the wheel of life so that he will have to be born again. But, because of his great desire for money, he will probably be in a position of poverty. This is his hell right here on Earth.

There may be a pull for service. There may be a pull for power. There may be a pull for fame or for position in life, like a dictator. There may be a pull for God, like Krishna. Many people said to him, "Maybe you are mad," and he said, "Yes, that's true. Many men are mad for gold and many men are mad for fame, many men are mad for power but too few men are mad for God."

You can hear the word reincarnation a million times, but it will be just a word until you can remember your past life, which you can do, and then it's a fact. Then you know; otherwise it's only conversation.

Buddha said a very beautiful thing, "Do not believe it because I have said it, do not believe it because you have read it, do not believe it because some sage has been inspired or thought he was inspired, but believe it when you know it in your heart," and then it becomes a thing of wisdom and no one can take it away from you.

There is an exercise to help you remember your past lives. For example, what was the first thing you did when you got out of bed this morning? Now think back, what was the next and the next and now think back over the day. What you are doing is exercising the subconscious because it's all in the subconscious. Then, think back to what you were doing ten years ago at this time and then try fifteen years ago and then try it in a past life and you can think back and you can do it. You may not do it right away but eventually you will get it and when you do you will never forget it and you will remember it as long as you live. It will be as clear to you as what happened this morning, and fifteen years from now it will still be that clear.

It's always in complete color. You may see an exaggeration in the size of fruit or flowers, but it's always in color and this is one of the esoteric ways you can tell it is real. Someone can put you under hypnosis or suggestion and take you back; then you may say this is just my imagination, but when you are face to face with your incarnation you know this is nobody but yourself.

The Rosicrucians and Theosophists teach a method for seeing your past lives. They put a candle on each side of the mirror, and as you stare into the mirror many times you will see your face change, but I don't approve of this because it may frighten you. Many people are terrified, and it's not a good thing to do until you have done it the other way which is the natural way. You will get one and then another and another. You won't get them all but you may get twenty or thirty or forty.

Many times as you develop spiritually you become more and more sensitive, and as you look at an individual you will see his face change one after the other very, very fast. I don't like this either because it becomes a parlor trick.

Many people who are able to remember several past lives find that the pattern of their lives repeats itself over and over again, so if you can go back far enough you can break that pattern.

We bring these same character traits and talents in with us lifetime after lifetime and keep doing the same things over and over again. For instance, suppose you have a talent for music. Your destiny for this incarnation may be to become a great musician, but you get a little lazy and don't work as hard as you could, so the next time around you will want to play but you won't have the ability. This is something that happens many times. If you are given a talent you must use it, or it will be taken away from you. The desire will remain but you will feel frustrated.

175. If you tell beginners in the Teaching about their past incarnations, this is very bad. Many people want me to tell them about their past lives but I say, "No, I want you to tell me and then I will check on it and tell you if you are correct. Then you know. Otherwise you only have my word and you haven't experienced it."

There is a story of an actress who was subsidizing herself between jobs by reading to this dear old lady who was slightly abstract and unbalanced; not mad, just vague. She was a sweet old lady and lived in this lovely hotel. I went for tea one day and she was off in her world, so we were talking about Marie Antoinette's necklace and the French Revolution, and in the middle of it she heard us mention

Marie Antoinette and she said, "Who did you say?" and we said, "Marie Antoinette" and she said, "Oh, charming lady. She was here yesterday for tea." This happens very frequently. You find thousands of Marie Antoinettes and hundreds of Cleopatras.

If someone has a problem, a hang-up, then we can make an exception and tell them. I remember this girl on Park Avenue who came to me with claustrophobia so bad that when she walked into an elevator she'd faint. She couldn't go to the theater or anywhere. She was in the music business and it meant she had to walk up 28 flights of stairs. She said, "This is terrible. I've been to doctors and psychiatrists and no one can help me. Can you help me?" I said, "Yes, if you can take an ugly shock." She said, "I'll try anything. Is it an electrical shock?" I said, "No, it's an emotional shock."

I could see what had caused this. It went back to an old Egyptian incarnation in which she was part of the Pharaoh's household, and when he died the whole family was taken into the pyramid with him and buried alive. When I told her this she broke out in a tremendous sweat and wept.

I said, "Now get your coat and hat. We're going down into Macy's basement and break this thing right now." The poor girl was in a state of shock and I had to hold onto her. We got down into the subbasement and I thought she was going to faint any minute, and suddenly the thing lifted and she never had it bother her again. In cases like this you are permitted to tell about the incarnation because this is an old fear that has hung over from many, many lifetimes.

176. As I have told you many times before, we are sum and substance of all our past lives. Your whole makeup is from your past lives, all your personality traits, everything.

As an example of this, the son of the English actress Gladys Cooper came to me one day and said, "You know, I was told in meditation that my mother was Queen Elizabeth," and I said, "Yes, this is true."

Gladys Cooper is a little bit of a woman, not at all pretentious. One night she came to the class and there must have been about eighty people there who did not know who she was. She isn't flashy or anything, but very quiet and very tiny. She walked in a little late and we were in the middle of the lesson, but every person in that room stood up right in the middle of the meeting. Here was the Queen. They felt this but they didn't know why they did it.

So I looked over at her son and winked and he winked back. She has that quality. Later we went to an opening and people bowed right and left, and there it is. She is still the Queen.

177. Incarnations alternate. One time you may be a woman and

the next time a man. Many times a man hater or a woman hater has to come back and experience that which they hate. So if a woman hates being a woman she will have to come back over and over as a woman until she learns to accept it and enjoy it; then she is free, and the same thing with a man. These are hang-ups that have to be worked out.

You come back in a body that is best suited to serve in. In any Teaching you are put into a family for karmic reasons so you can work out this karma. The main thing is not to be resentful. Just say, this is my karma and I've got to work it out, and the moment you take this attitude your resentments are gone.

There was a woman I knew in New York who was completely paralyzed with arthritis. She couldn't move her hands. She couldn't feed herself, nothing. The poor thing was in a hotel, and she couldn't get up or out or anything, so four or five of our group went and took care of her, fed her and bathed her for about three weeks, and then she was up and moving.

What had happened was that she was married to a very handsome, romantic Hungarian. Her best friend was fat while this woman was very attractive, but her husband fell in love with her friend and just walked out on her, and she was so resentful of the girl that it brought on this paralysis. I told her, "You have to get rid of this resentment or you'll never get well until you do." So she prayed and prayed and one day she said, "I'm through with all this," and then she began to get well. Today she is just fine.

Frustration and resentment can cause many illnesses, and it's been said this is oftentimes a cause of cancer.

Alternation of incarnation also means you may skip a cycle. You may remain for a longer period of time in the Subtle World after death.

This is how it works. The Dalai Lama or the Tashi Lama, the moment He dies, in a split second He is reborn because He is a very high consciousness. This is true of very high souls. Now the other people are in a different category. They may have to rest for a period of time in order to adjust to another rebirth, to develop on the subtle plane before they come back again. They may skip a couple of lifetimes or they may come back every time until they know exactly what they are doing.

For instance, in the Teaching They ask, "Why are we here? What is our purpose?" It is to learn to be aware of the difficulties of all people, to be available to all people, to create an actual Brotherhood that functions in the world. This is the whole purpose of our being here and when we know this, then our job will bring us back time after time after time much faster, because we are needed for this work.

Whatever baggage of wisdom we take over with us we use there, and if we go over as a stupid or narrow person we cannot expect to come back brilliant, so it's a continuation of the search for wisdom, and when we have added more we are ready for rebirth to see if we can make it in that life.

178. The average length of time between lifetimes for people not in the Teachings is 700 years. The higher the evolution of the individual the faster they are brought back. Like the Dalai Lama who is reborn within a split second.

This reminds me of the story of this young man out in San Francisco who came and asked to become a disciple. He told me he had taken LSD two or three years ago. "But," he said, "I'm never going to take it again because it brought me this realization; I saw the whole karmic pattern of birth and death, birth and death and how damn hopeless it was. It seemed so hopeless I wanted to go out and destroy myself. I knew I was on that wheel of karma and from that moment I decided I was going to get off somehow. I didn't know how but I had to find a solution. That's how I came into the Teaching. My desperation brought me to it." He said, "I've talked to many people and they have this same vision of hopelessness."

This is the karma of these people who wait 700 years and then come back to do the same stupid things over and over again. That's the tragic part; over and over and over again. This is what Buddha taught, from house to house of flesh, born on that wheel to live and die and be born and live and die until you learn to get off.

The greatest thing in the world is to have wisdom. Not the wisdom of books but the wisdom of the law of cosmos and nature. To know why we are alive, what we are doing here, what we are preparing for, what's happening next. This is why the churches and schools have failed. This is why we are having riots in the colleges [the 1960's], because basically there is a great need to change.

I think I told you about the man who dropped the first bomb on Hiroshima. He wrote to his father and said, "I may die tomorrow. I have graduated from college with my masters degree but I don't know how to die." This is true of many people. They are completely unprepared. They are filled with fears and insecurity. But when you know that actually this whole thing is a development of spirit, and the moment you get off that wheel your whole karmic pattern will change, then you will be free. Until then you are tied to being reborn every 700 years over and over again.

179. "In the book, *The Mahatma Letters,* they say there is a circle or cycle and man starts out as pure spirit and descends into matter and

then works his way up to spirituality again. Are the beginning and the end the same?"

No, the beginning and the end are never the same. Let's take the face of a clock and visualize the twelve and three and six and nine. Now, at twelve o'clock the seed of the spirit comes into the soul and this soul then enters into a physical body and reincarnates and reincarnates through various lives and experiences, moving counterclockwise into more and more gross matter. And people will remain in these various experiences and never move on until they realize why they are here and how to fall off the wheel of birth, life and death. They just keep doing the same things over and over again because this is karma at work, the law of cause and effect, until one day they get damn good and sick of it and say, what is wrong with me? What am I doing that is causing all this pain? The minute they see all this as a result of their own actions, their karma changes. When they become aware of karma, then they can work it out through birth, life and death and through sacrifice and work for humanity.

We have all gone through incarnations of being Jewish, being colored, being Arab, being everything, and you come out of it understanding these people and their problems and you don't condemn them for their actions because you too have done what they are doing now. When you realize your incarnations you don't condemn anyone for anything because again this is the Christ principle, "Judge not lest ye be judged." It's also a principle in Buddhism, in Zoroastrianism and Judaism. In all these scriptures they give hints, telling us not to involve ourselves in the karma of other people by condemning them, so what you do is let them go and know this is something they are working out. It may be obnoxious to you but you look at these individuals as being blind.

As Christ said, "They have eyes and they see not, they have ears and they hear not." This is exactly what He was talking about. If a blind man or woman walked into you on the street, you wouldn't think anything of it. You'd say, this man is blind, and you'd excuse him and bless him and help him. So if you can see all people in this way and say, "They are blind, therefore they cannot see what they are doing; I forgive them for whatever it is," then you release yourself from all that karma and you are free.

For instance, we have been cheats and liars and murderers and everything else because we have gone through all these cycles and learned our lessons and stopped doing these things. Finally, we come as a little child, pure of heart, no guile, no trickery but sincere and honest and there it is, but you have to go through the fire in order to obtain this thing of spirit. You have to live in the world but not be of it in order to leave it. This is the great trick: that nothing touches you.

In the end this seed of the spirit is pure and sophisticated, but wise.

180. In the law of reincarnation there is no retrogression. A chela who comes from another planet to work here and then loses his chelaship does not lose all the accumulations he has acquired, but he stands still for a certain period of time and later moves on again. When that happens another individual is given that whole essence and his development is speeded up with that knowledge. The chela was not sent to Earth to learn that lesson but he has free will to make mistakes. Always remember that the free will of man plays a most important role. One of the great rules of the Mahatmas is to never dominate another person. All wars and dissention are caused by the domination of one person over another. This is wrong.

The knowledge you have brought in from another planet to this one is blocked because it would destroy you. It's too much. For instance, how would you describe infinity? You know what the word is and you have some vague idea that it's an abstraction, but do you understand it? Or if someone said, what is fifty billion dollars? You know it in figures, but the human mind can't conceive what it actually is. Or can you describe God? You can't do it. In the East they won't even attempt to try, because it is so far beyond the human consciousness.

If you came in with this complete knowledge and were born into a family of Earthlings, how would you fit into that life? You'd go crazy; so you are blocked, except that certain essences will come out and there will be certain traces of knowledge. For instance, many children have an inborn knowledge of reincarnation. They say, I know I've lived before.

Earlier I told you the story of the little three-year-old girl in Texas who remembered having been the Dalai Lama's mother (para. 122). This is only one example of children who bring in this knowledge with them. There are many more.

181. Knowing your past lives can lead to problems, especially if you have had a high position or have been very important. You become attached to this and then it becomes very hard to adjust in this life.

There is a rather tragic yet amusing story about a man in New York. He called me one day and asked me to come over. He said he was suffering from a great feeling of guilt because he was certain he had been Nero in another life. So I went over to see him and it was obvious that he wasn't Nero and never had been. I said, "No, this is not your past life at all. You have never been Nero." He almost cried. He said, "I'm only an insignificant little barber and this was the only thing that made me feel important. Now you've ruined it." I said,

"Well, if you want to imagine that you are Nero, go right ahead."

The personality we have now is a condensation of all of our past lives. Many times we bring in certain tendencies from the past such as laziness or a weak will, and if we know what they are we can do something about it. Many times it's a very fine thing we bring in, like the child who at seven is conducting an orchestra.

These children are New Agers, and they have full knowledge of who they are and where they are going. They can give you an explanation of reincarnation and karma that will make your hair stand on end. They know it. They have brought it in with them. They have a fantastic ability to read back into their past lives. In California we had a group of children who wanted to have a class in yoga and so we met with them. When we meditated we told them to ask, "Who am I, what am I here for, what is my purpose?" Afterward it was like listening to seventy-year-olds who had been studying this all their lives. These children knew their path and what they were to do, much more than many adults.

One little girl of nine said, "I was a dancer in a former life. I saw this in meditation: I didn't want to have children because it would ruin my career, so in this life I must marry early and have a family to make up for this selfishness."

These children are so close to this recall. They are very open, and they remember until they are about seven or eight, and then they lose it because people say no, that's not the way it is at all. In the school in Texas the children were shown a picture of my Guru, Nicholas Roerich. A little child of about four said, "Teacher, this is a man of light." They know. They have this pure observation. You cannot fool them.

Now there are many people in all walks of life who are looking for answers. Store clerks, taxi drivers, students, the young people, and many others are all asking the same questions, "Why are we here, what are we working out, what is our purpose?"

Of course we are here to work towards our spiritual development and to get wisdom, and when we have this wisdom we are to put it to work in teaching, in building, in medicine, in science, in art, in music, and in all of these forms. This is what we are to do. This is why we are here. We are to use our wisdom to make this a better world.

182. By the sacrifice of Joan of Arc—when she would not admit to the Chruch that the voices she heard were of the devil—she reincarnated as HPB, and then Blavatsky, by her sacrifice, reincarnated as a Greek monk in Syria. It is said that Jesus has also returned to incarnation in Syria, and at the time of the death of Pope Pius it

was predicted one of the two would become the next Pope.

As you know, the law of reincarnation and the law of karma was struck out in 555 A.D. and this Pope was to bring those laws back into focus where they should be and put the responsibility on the people instead of the Church. But you know what happened. They became chauvinistic and had to have an Italian. If you remember, the smoke went up white and then it went black and then white. Pope Pius was actually the beginning of the end of the Catholic Church and now look at it; it's collapsing all over the place.

It's good that the priests and nuns are marrying. There is no reason why they shouldn't. In the Greek churches they are allowed to marry and have families, and they are the mystics. We are going through a whole revolution of everything. It's the end of all this control over people and it's wonderful.

183. Did people reincarnate on the Earth from the sun? No, the sun is not populated. It is merely a source of energy, a storehouse of energy, a thing of consciousness. It is not gaseous as the scientists tell us. They merely assume the sun is gaseous.

Scientists are frequently wrong. Fifty years ago if you would have said, pictures will come into my house through a screen without wires, they would have said you were nuts. Many years ago Tesla said there was energy around all matter and that matter is energy and they laughed at him, but Einstein came along and proved him to be right.

Science is still limited. To quote Aldous Huxley, "The only way they're ever going to overcome their limitations is through metaphysics," which means "that which is beyond science (or physics)." The Mahatmas are not limited. They have straight knowledge. They know.

Thousands of years ago in the Upanishads and Vedas they speak constantly of the atom. This is why in India they can levitate, because they know how to reverse the atoms in their body and defy the law of gravity; in the same way they do the rope trick, where they make a rope go straight up in the air, climb up and disappear.

Speaking of disappearing, you can try putting on the cloak of invisibility. This is a thing that anyone can do because it's a way of thinking. You are visible to other people, but to the person you don't want to see you, you are invisible.

I tested this one time coming from Long Island. I was with this charming girl, a writer, who was a little light minded. She would say, "Well, I have to have proof." She was skeptical of everything. We were riding along and she said, "This stupid Long Island Railroad, I'd really like to give them a good screwing." And I said, "Well, why don't you. Take the money in your hand but don't show it to the conductor. Don't move, don't look at it, and think of making yourself completely invisible—you are not here." So she sat there and didn't move a muscle. She sat across from me and looked at me. The conductor came by and took everybody's ticket and passed her by. He couldn't see her. He walked all the way down the car and back again. He knew there was something wrong. He went through that car eleven times looking for that missing person but he couldn't see her. She rode all the way into the station with the money in her hand.

Personality and Individuality

184. I am often asked to explain the difference between the personality and individuality. The individuality is the essence of the soul. It's the complete unity of the monad.

The personality, which is made up of charm, sincerity, love, intelligence, wisdom, etc., is built with each lifetime. You keep building it bigger and stronger and finer and you're making your vehicle better, or worse, whichever. All of these things become part of the individuality. Esoterically, the words monad and individuality are synonymous.

The sum and substance of all you are, of all your personalities from all your past lives and what you have done with them, the sum of spirit, soul, and mind; all of it put together is the individuality.

Now many people become frightened of losing their personality by being overshadowed by a Mahatma or Guru. You don't lose, you gain; you grow stronger. Like my Guru, who gave me more than I ever had or would have had. He opened up many things for me. Actually, everything I am or ever will be I owe to my Guru and his overshadowing me. I couldn't ask for a greater blessing.

185. From the source of your spirit and soul many times a particular dominant feature from the personality of a former life will come to the surface.

Everything you have ever been on the planet you came from before coming to Earth—like Venus and Jupiter, which are two of the highest planets in the solar system—is also part of you. The total monad goes all the way back. Originally you came from pure spirit.

Many people say, why wasn't I born a man or why wasn't I born a woman? It's because the body you have now is equipped for the job you are doing at this particular time. It's not karmic when you are in the Teaching. When you are not in the Teaching, it's karmic.

186. The monad is that immortal part of man, the seed of the spirit, which reincarnates from lifetime to lifetime. It is not the personality. Basically it's the individuality or the soul, that portion of the spirit that creates itself. It's the wholeness of one; the creation of the spirit.

During each lifetime, the monad either accumulates or it sleeps. The accumulations are added to the monad as you go along from lifetime to lifetime, and this draws you closer and closer to the Lord of that particular planet on which you are working.

It works on the same principle as putting money in the bank and getting your interest. You may go three years and not deposit anything, and then you may deposit a large amount. It's the same with life. You may have one lifetime and put very little into it, so the next one you make up for that. There is no retrogression, but karma must be worked out. You cannot lose what you have in spirit. Even if a disciple breaks, they cannot retrogress, thank God. They can incur very bad karma, but they will always keep what they have even if they don't use it in that lifetime.

There are exceptions like Mr. X., and Mr. Y., who violated a shrine. It may be a manvantara before they get a chance to come back again. They tore down two shrines in the Roerich Institute: the Shrine of St. Sergius and the Shrine of Buddha. In these two shrines I had my initiation, half in one and half in the other. To violate any religious thing is bad enough if you don't know what you are doing, but they knew. This is the most heinous crime you can commit, even worse than any kind of murder, because this is a violation of God.

This is why They always warn us, if you don't know about somebody's philosophy or religion, never tear it apart. This is also a violation. They are what they are for a reason. Their God is their God and it's none of our business how they worship or what they do, unless they come to us for instruction and help. If they don't, we must not force our God on them. As the Teachings say, "Not by my God, but by thy God."

God Consciousness

187. God Consciousness is the idea of becoming one with all the laws of nature. Buddha said that he entered into the dead body of

a jackass, and had the whole feeling of this jackass; and he entered into the dead body of a bird; into the dead body of a pig, and he felt the whole thing of these different animals.

The idea is: when you can be as a mirror and reflect the other person into you, this is being one with God. Then you can see their point of view and understand their problems and can help them, but unless you have that ability you are helpless. It's being impersonal and loving people, and then when they talk to you, you know exactly what is going on in their mind and in their heart. This is being one with God.

188. The fastest way to God Consciousness is through healing. We can talk and discuss and exchange ideas with someone endlessly, but the fastest way is to heal them. This is the great unseen gift. Something magic happens and they are never the same again. They will say, we have experienced this. We know it. Otherwise it is only conversation. When it becomes an experience, no one can take it away from you and no one can talk you out of it, because you know it in your heart.

189. Many Teachers, like Krishnamurti, say you have God Consciousness within you and all you have to do is bring it out. But how do you do that? You have to learn to do it and it's a slow process. It's actually blood, sweat and tears to make it operate and function, because we are living in a world of matter. It becomes easier if you have your chosen image before you. And to achieve this, what you do is take your personal concept of the image of God, whatever it may be, and then repeat very simply this prayer of the heart, "May I through my heart see the image of Thy reflection." If you continue to use this prayer over and over, suddenly the image will appear and will remain forever and ever, so be sure you are ready to live with that image for the rest of your life.

190. Just as all religions are one, so we should be one with all the laws of nature. This is a very wonderful thing to try: sit and concentrate on a flower and continue to concentrate and suddenly your whole heartbeat and your whole essence becomes that flower for a moment, or try being one with a tree or plant. It will only be for a couple of minutes but you and the object you're concentrating on will be one during that time. It's a very beautiful experience and something everyone can do but very few people do it.

Or, another thing you can do is go out into the park or anywhere the butterflies fly and hold out your hand and call, "Butterfly come," and they will come to you. What you are actually doing is ionizing the air around you and they lose their fear that you will hurt them. They will land on your hand and stay until you tell them to go. Of course, if you are destructive they will not land. What happens is, that with your heart element you reach out and touch the heart element of the butterfly or bird or animal and at that moment you are one with it and all fear is released. You can even do this to a gentleman butterfly who is chasing a lady butterfly with no good intentions. He will actually stop his flight and land on your hand.

When man goes out into the country and close to nature he learns the secret laws of nature by being a part of it and becoming one with it. As Swami Bodinanda used to say, "There are sermons in the stones. There is wisdom in the brook, and wisdom in the trees if we can but hear it." Now when we can be still, as Christ said, "Be still and know that you are one with God," then you have it.

There is a beautiful story in the book *Siddhartha,* called "The Song of Life," in which he tells of a man who crosses the river as a young man and goes through all these experiences and gets entangled with karma and maya. He makes a fortune, marries and has a family, and then he comes back across the river as an old man and he realizes the river is the song of nature, and from this he gains great cosmic wisdom and he stays on as the man who ferries the boat back and forth across the river.

190. Some people can't wait to get across the river and some people think the river is put there to hinder them, but very few people ever pause and listen to what the river has to say. When we can quiet ourselves to the point where we can hear the voice of nature, then we will have a cosmic understanding of nature, and be one with it instead of being one amongst it.

The whole idea of being in the Teaching is to be a mirror and reflect the concepts of the other person on their level. When you can say, "Not by my God but by thy God," then you are communing with the nature of the individual. You are the mirror and you are the reflection. It's from the heart and not by words, and the heart can say volumes and the lips very little.

191. All legends are based on truth. Your Greek gods and goddesses were actually the essence of people who knew cosmic law and could handle cosmic law. There are forces in nature than can be handled; for instance, your Indians can produce rain any time they want. This is not fiction. They do it. If we were more in tune with nature, we too could do all these things, but we are out of that rhythm. We are so far out of it we are not working with nature at all. This is the idea of cosmic law and when you work with it, nature and cosmic law are one and the same.

192. Plato's twin soul concept is the idea of the development of the twin soul within man himself. When you have come to a perfect

balance of the two, the male and the female, then you have found the twin soul, but man must find that balance within himself. You see, he always looks for it outside himself, in other people, but when we have the refinement of the female and the masculinity of the male put together in a constructive way, then you have this union with God within yourself.

Without this union people are always searching for something outside. This fulfillment is God Consciousness and basically this is what every soul is seeking; that consciousness that will make them complete within themselves. They go around on this wheel of karma and they're looking for it out here in all of this illusion and maya, when all the time it's right here inside.

It's the old story of the bluebird: the German who went all over the world looking for a bluebird, and when he came back he found it right in his own backyard.

There was a man who wanted to see God. He said, if I could see God and know that he exists, I would be fulfilled. So he went to the Archbishop of Canterbury in England and asked, and the Archbishop said, no, he had never seen God but he knew a great deal about God. Then he went to the Pope in Rome and asked and he said, no, he had never seen God but he knew all about the way to do it. Then he went to the Dalai Lama and He said, no, He had never seen God but He knew all the traditions and prayers.

So finally he went to Simla up in the mountains in India and on the road he met a monk and asked, "Have you seen God?" And the monk looked at him and said, "Yes, I always see God." So the man said, "Tell me, how do you see him?" The monk said, "Go up to the top of the mountain and there you will find a temple, climb to the roof and clear away the debris and you will see God." The man hurried up the mountain, climbed to the roof of the temple, cleared away the debris and there was a shining surface. He looked and saw his own reflection.

This is what Christ meant when he said, "Be still and know that I am God." And when you get a glimpse of the God within yourself, you've got it, just like that. This is why in the East, when they bow to you with hands together touching the forehead, they mean, I bow to the God within you. As Buddha said, "Men cry out and pray for God Consciousness, but it is within you and all you have to do is reach out and touch it and it is yours forever and ever beyond the wildest dreams of man." It's peace and contentment because you have an understanding of yourself, and this is within all people.

193. As we have said many times, selflessness is one of the fastest ways to God Consciousness. The moment you see anyone in difficulty, go and help them, or it may be a simple thing like picking

up after someone around your home. Many times people are very careless and throw things around. Go and pick it up and say this is part of my unselfishness. Pick it up and put it away and don't say anything. The thing is, you know this is going to help them and it's going to make you feel better, too. Instead of feeling imposed upon, you say, this is my opportunity to grow. It's a great opportunity because this thing of service is the great unseen gift that is all around us. Too few people are aware of it, but once you can utilize it you have a golden key beyond all the wildest dreams of mankind. You have the key to real contentment, the key to real love, to understanding and selflessness. "I think not of myself but of others." "I think not of my time but of others," and the moment you do you will not feel like a martyr, but you will feel, "This is my chance to serve." How else can we serve but to serve other people.

You see, God is an abstraction. He is not a man with a big stick on a throne, so we are his hands and feet and eyes and ears. I told you about the two Canadian boys who were walking past a house one day and they heard the people inside praying for bread. So they thought they would play a funny joke on them. They went to a store and bought several loaves of bread and went back and threw them in the window. They were telling me about it and they thought it was a very amusing joke. I said, "Actually, you were the servant of the Lord because you answered their prayers."

In India the people take care of their Teachers and supply them with food and transportation or whatever needs they may have. It is the same with Vedanta. The monks own nothing, not even a watch to tell time. They give up their name and call themselves Asachananda. Ananda means brother. Everything must be offered to them, otherwise they never ask for anything.

One Christmas a group of us wanted to give Swami Bodhananda, who was eighty-three a present. We knew he wouldn't accept money so we asked in meditation and were told that he needed warm blankets and a pillow and a warm meditation shawl because he was old.

We asked the housekeeper and she said, "I am so glad you asked. I couldn't tell anyone because he would be displeased." They feel that if God wants them to have it, God will send it. They know God will use another individual to provide these things, so they never thank the individual; they thank God, which is the proper thing to do.

194. Starr Daly found his Guru in prison. His Guru had killed his own wife and yet he died in a state of Samadhi, which is the highest state of consciousness that can be attained. He had asked for forgiveness in his heart, sincerely, and he was forgiven.

Reams of words have been written about Starr Daly. In his book,

Stone Walls Do Not A Prison Make, he tells of how he spent most of his life in prison. I knew him and he told me he was a pretty ugly person and had spent much of his time in solitary confinement.

One day they strung him up by the hands so that just the tips of his toes barely touched the floor. They left him there for three days and suddenly he went into God Consciousness and became clairvoyant. He tells about it in his book. He said, "It was cold. It was damp." He remembers it because his Teacher had said, "Whatever it is, wherever you are, you can make it into something else." So he said, "The room was cold. I asked that it be warm. I visualized a stove and a fireplace. I visualized it furnished with beautiful furniture and paintings and I had sunlight coming in." And he said, "I did this all in my mind because it was a black cell," and he said, "Suddenly, I reached a saturation level, I let go and had a complete realization. It changed my whole life."

When they let him out, he went to the warden and said, "My whole life has changed. I want to preach on Sunday." They roared with laughter, "The worst convict in the prison and you want to preach. What are you going to teach them?" He said, "No, I mean it. I have a message and I want to do this." When he got up before all those prisoners they laughed and jeered, but he went right on talking and suddenly they quieted down and every Sunday after that he was their minister.

He and his Guru had been cell mates, and his Guru had taught him all these things. Of course being strung up by your thumbs is an artificial means of attaining clairvoyance, so don't try it in your cellar.

When we talked he told me, "Mr. H., the secret of this whole thing is meditation, meditation and more meditation."

And in his book, he said, "When I was in prison I thought I was confined, but then I realized I was released and I realized that thousands and thousands of people are walking around prisoners of their fears and hate and prejudice." He said, "These are terrible prisons. They are much worse than prison bars."

When he was finally released from prison, he lectured all over the United States and Canada and wrote many books. He really was a terrific person.

195. Buddha attained enlightenment first and then He gave it to others. You cannot give enlightenment to others if you don't have it yourself. But, when you have a light burning in your soul and with that light you can set another soul on fire, then you have it. Otherwise, you are a parrot reciting.

Buddha was a royal prince. He gave up a kingdom for an even greater kingdom. As Christ said, "If you will give up houses and mothers and fathers and brothers and sisters, I will give you more houses and mothers and fathers and brothers and sisters.'' All the Avatars taught the same thing, but Buddha was the only one who taught the release from the wheel of birth and death and for this he went to Nirvana.

There is a beautiful story about a holy man who was lecturing to his disciples and he said, ''I will tell you ten words and with these words you can escape your karma, and if you will repeat them just before you pass over you will not have to come back to Earth, but if you tell anyone else they will escape their karma and you will have to come back in their place.'' There were fifteen monks who heard this. Fourteen thought, this is a wonderful piece of information, but the one remaining monk went out into the street and told everyone he met about the ten words. The holy man said, ''There is my one disciple. He was willing to take on the karma of strangers in order that they be released through this knowledge.''

Now who had enlightenment, the people who were holding it for themselves or the one who was willing to give it away? Buddha released everything one hundred percent, but not many are willing to do this. You too can escape your karma if you plunge into this thing and give everything you have to it.

196. I am often asked about Nirvana. Let me try to explain in this way. Imagine yourself sitting on top of a train where you can see into the future, into the past, and that which is the present. This is the whole idea of clairvoyance, because you're seeing in three dimensions. When you're using the conscious mind it's like looking out of the window of the train, but when you are in control of your subconscious mind or using straight knowledge you're seeing the future, the present and the past all in one. Nirvana goes way beyond that.

Actually, Nirvana cannot be visualized. It's impossible for the human mind to conceive it. It's like the word God; you can't define the word. In the East they won't even mention the word God because it is so far beyond the ability of man to conceive. Nirvana is the same idea.

Buddha is the only Avatar who made Nirvana. He has reached that state of God Consciousness in which there is no return to being an individual, but his whole essence and seed of the spirit has become one with God.

He discovered the secret of falling off the wheel of karma, of not being torn by desire or hunger or cold or loneliness, or the desire to be with people, or fame or fortune or power. All of these things He rose above and by completely eliminating them, He obtained Nirvana.

He's up on the seventh round, there by Himself waiting for the rest of humanity to move up.

Buddha came from Jupiter as Vishnu and after thirteen incarnations ended up as Buddha. Again we have this thirteen. The last Dalai Lama was the thirteenth Dalai Lama and the last Pope in the true sense of the word was the thirteenth Pope. Thirteen is not an unlucky number. This is superstition. Thirteen in numerology is four and that is a very high spiritual number.

God

197. Letter No. 10 in *The Mahatma Letters* is the letter on God in which the Mahatmas say They do not believe in God as an individual but as an impersonal consciousness of Brahman. They do not believe in a personal God because God is infinite, so therefore he cannot be personal.

What we call God is the great wisdom, the great intelligence that exists and holds the whole planetary system together. It is the divine principle in wisdom, the immutable law, so therefore it cannot be a personality.

So many churches teach that God is a man sitting on a golden throne with a big stick. They say that God made man in His image, then man turned around and made God in his. This is unfortunate because it makes God finite when in fact He is infinite. In the East the concept of God is so great they will not even try to define or describe Him, because they say it's beyond the human mind to comprehend. You can't possibly describe Him, because the minute you put it into words you limit it, and how can you limit something that is limitless?

Very often in trying to put this concept into words, there is no language for it. This is why many times in the East, when a disciple has developed to a certain level, the teaching is given silently by the Guru from the heart to the heart, and this is the most perfect form of the teaching. There are no misunderstandings, no misinterpretations whatsoever, because it's a cosmic thing.

In many churches they teach that God is a jealous God and He will punish you for your sins. This is nonsense. How could a divine image that is so great be punishing people? Instead of saying we are paying for our karma, they blame it on God. It's the same as saying that Christ died for our sins. It's very comfortable to put the entire load on Him, but this is only an excuse to blame someone else when actually we make our own quality, our own karma, and nobody is at fault but us.

198. There is no limitation on the concept of God, only the limitation we put on it. In the same way, we also limit ourselves. When we say we can't do it, it means we're too lazy to do it or we don't have enough confidence in ourselves to do it, or we don't want to do it.

As God is everything there is no good and there is no evil. It's all one but what we see or what we put into it is what makes it good or evil. One person may do something that we consider evil or bad, but that may be an experience they have to go through. We may have already gone through it a couple thousand years ago. As Christ said, "Judge not lest ye be judged." Everything is experience. If you put your hand in the fire you will be burned and you don't do it again. If you do you're stupid, and you deserve to be burned.

One day this man and I were talking and he was talking of God as a personality and I said, "Oh no, God is an abstraction and is not a personality at all," and he said, "Oh, Mr. H., my brother is a Jesuit priest, and my parish priest teaches that God is a personality." I said, "Well, you may think that if you like but it's not true." He said, "I'll ask my brother." I said, "Fine, you do that and then tell me what he said, I'll be very interested."

So the following week he came back and said, "You've upset my apple cart. I told my brother what you said, and he said, 'The gentleman is right. God is an abstraction.' I was horrified because my priest always led me to believe that God was a personality. My brother said, 'Did he ever tell you that?' and I said, 'No, but I assumed.' My brother said, 'Go back and talk to your priest because to assume a thing is very wrong.'" So he said, "I went to my priest and he said, 'No, I never told you that, but if people are stupid enough to think that God is a personality many times it is easier to control them than if they believe God is an abstraction.'" This is an example of working with masses of people. Many times a great truth is a dangerous thing to tell. It could be distorted and misused.

199. Since God is an abstraction, He has no hands nor feet nor lips nor eyes. We are his lips, his hands, his eyes, his brain and therefore we are the servants of God and do his work. The majority of people reverse it and want God to do everything for them. You should say, "May I serve you?"

There is a story of this Maharaja who went to the monks at a nearby monastery and said, "If ever you need money come and see me and I will give it to you." So hard times fell on the monastery and they sent one of the monks to the Maharaja. The king was praying, but the majordomo said, "Go right in. He'll be delighted to see you."

So the monk went in and he heard the king praying, "Oh God, give me more lands. Oh God, give me greater armies, give me more taxes from the people, more grain, more power." When the king came out the majordomo said, ". . . the monk has been here but left." The king said, "Take a horse and go and bring him back." When the monk came in the king said, "It's obvious you came for help. What is it you want?" The monk said, "Yes, I came to ask a king for help but instead I found a beggar, and I cannot accept anything from a beggar."

Speaking of monks, there is a wonderful old saying we've put up on one of the doors at the Ashram. It is from one of the ancient monasteries of about the year 1500 and it says, "If any monk in this monastery is dissatisfied he is only to approach us and explain his views because this may be God speaking through him and we may learn something from him, but if he proves to be gossipy, tiresome and a nuisance let it be explained to him he must depart. If he does not do so, two stout monks will accompany him to the door."

200. You have to want God or you're never going to find Him. If you have a great need for God such as a great hunger, or you're terribly poor or ill, then you will find Him, but where there is no great need most people don't look for Him. They are quite content to go along and say, "Christ died for our sins, so why should I bother?" and they only have a bowing acquaintance with the Lord. I've often said, some people kneel on one knee, some bow their heads, but in the East they touch their forehead to the dust, and there is a difference. We cannot be proud and go to the Lord; we have to go in complete humbleness.

201. As you all know the birthplace of the United Nations is San Francisco. A few years ago [1955] on the anniversary of its founding there was a week-long series of meetings there. We got together with Dr. Pettipher and tried to find a place for meditation and prayer that we could use during that week. We went to the Scottish Rite and asked for the use of their auditorium on Van Ness Avenue and every day between ten o'clock in the morning and three o'clock in the afternoon, every religion in the world came in and for forty-five minutes spoke on their form of God, the brotherhood of man and world peace. Then for the next fifteen minutes we all meditated on world peace. We had Moslem, Buddhist, Hindu, all the religions. The only one that didn't come was the Roman Catholic. The Bishop refused, saying they do not recognize any other religion and therefore could not participate. But all the other religions were represented; the Mormons, even an Islamic group called the Sufi. It

was a tremendous, wonderful thing; the first time in the history of the world that all religions spoke from the same podium on the same subject in the same harmony. These were diversified people working together. This was so powerful that at night a great white light could be seen over the hall, going right up into the sky.

One of the men who spoke was a Moslem priest, a real man of God. His speech was fiery and very, very wonderful, and he said, "God is like the impressario of an orchestra and He must be the only one. Then there is the first violin and the second and so on." And then he said, "God must come first, even before my wife, my children or my country; first must come the Lord." Afterward I went to him and thanked him and said, "You are a great man of God and I admire you very much." And he said, "No, Mr. H., I'm not a man of God—yet. I am trying to be but you see I am only a Moslem priest, therefore I am only a small slice of God, but when I have fulfilled my mission here and I have taken care of my wife and family, I will go to India and I shall go up into the hills and then I shall bow to God in all forms and only then shall I be a man of God."

If we are only one religion then we are only a small section of the whole, but if we can embrace God in every shape and form then we are completely one with the whole and only then. But if we have prejudice, if we say my group is right and everybody else is wrong, you cannot move beyond that point and you are stuck with that particular karma.

202. Many people say, oh yes, I believe in Mahatmas, but they don't expect to ever see one, and when they do it's a terrific shock because they don't actually believe.

The same is true in churches. The ministers and priests talk about God and all of these things but they don't really believe. One day I was riding on the train with these two ministers and they were talking and one said, "We need a new roof for the church." And the other one said, "We could have a bazaar or a dinner." Then they asked me, "What would you do?" I said, "I'd ask God." They were operating on the mental level and not from the heart. How can they teach if they don't believe? It's the blind leading the blind.

I was talking to a woman who spends all her time in a wheelchair. She's a Quaker and completely devoted to prayer and God and all this sort of thing, and yet her spine was so bad she couldn't get out of bed without help. I said to her, "I know a group of people who do healing through prayer. Would you like to be put on the list? I'm sure they could help you." She said, "I don't believe in that kind of prayer." They profess one thing but practice another. They really don't believe.

Mother of the World

203. As God is the masculine principle in the Universe, so The Mother of the World is the feminine principle. In India she is called Kali; in China, Quan Yin; in Japan, Quo Yu; and in Egypt, the Mother is Isis.

Some years ago I knew this young lawyer in New York City who was being sent to India by the State Department to do some very important work. A few days before he was to go, he began running a temperature of 103°. He called and said, "R., would you come and help me get this fever down?" We went and did this count down on fever and by ten it was gone. He was weak and so I said, "Tomorrow I want you to stay in bed. I'll come over and bring your breakfast and stay to get your lunch."

The next morning when I saw him he said, "R., what is the Mother of the World?" I explained and he said, "I'm Greek Orthodox and we know about the Virgin, but last night I woke up and I saw a figure and it was veiled with a jeweled veil and all I could see were the lips and the chin and she was all in beautiful blue and silver and she spoke to me and said...". I interrupted him, "Don't repeat it. This is personal and just for you. Never repeat it to another human being unless it's your Guru and I'm not." He said, "Could this be a hallucination as a result of my fever?" And I said, "Well, if there is any doubt, ask for it to appear again and give you the same message."

The next morning he told me the same thing happened. He said, "Suddenly it was like a shifting of silver light and she appeared in the room so clearly that I could see the outline of her feet, her hands, everything, and she gave me the same message."

I said, "This is a very wonderful thing because you are going on a mission to India which is very important." I got him off on the plane and six months later he came back and I saw him again. I said, "Did anything happen on your mission that related to the Mother of the World?" He said, "What Mother of the World?" And I said, "Your vision." He said, "What vision?" I said, "The one you had two nights in a row." He said, "I don't recall." It was completely wiped out of his memory. His ego had become so involved in what he was doing he forgot the whole thing. He had been given a responsibility but he didn't want it.

The Mother of the World is the mother of the entire Cosmos. It's the female concept. When we speak of God we say He, which is the male concept, but the two are actually indistinguishable. God or Brahman is one gender but in our language we speak of he and she. It's the combination of the twin element which is both mother and father, masculine and feminine. It belongs to the entire Cosmos and can take any form.

St. Sergius had an experience in which he actually saw a formation representing God and his hair turned white overnight. His disciple who was with him almost died.

Isis is the representation of cosmic knowledge and Isis is always veiled. You can only penetrate through the veil a little, until you have your fourth initiation and then the veil is lifted. This is the beginning of the opening of your consciousness. It's both symbolic and actual. When the veil is lifted you approach closer and closer to Truth.

Let me explain it another way. When the Mahatmas appear, a lot of people, including those who have been in the Teaching a long time, are skeptical that this can happen and until it happens to them it is only conversation. When it happens to you, my God, what a tremendous revelation, and you are no longer the person you were before, but this takes densifying their vibration and lifting yours, otherwise you couldn't take it. It would blast you to pieces. This is what happened to St. Sergius. The human body is actually a hindrance to the spirit.

Wisdom

204. During WWII there were three men completely cut off and surrounded by the enemy. The officer said, "Does anyone here know how to pray?" One soldier said, "Yes, when I was a little boy, I remember saying, 'Now I lay me down to sleep.' " So the officer said, "Use it and try to get some help for us." He did and they were rescued—on that prayer.

It doesn't matter what the words are. It doesn't have to be a great ritual in a great cathedral. It's in your heart, and when you ask you will receive. As Christ said, "Ask and you shall receive. Knock and the door shall be opened unto you." We can stand in front of the door forever and if we don't ask, nothing will happen. But this is our right, our heritage, our privilege to ask, to demand that the door to spiritual consciousness be opened to us, so that we may become attuned to the Universe or Cosmos or God or whatever you want to call it.

Many times you will have to search for it and even fight for it, and oftentimes beat your head against the door, but the search is worth every effort because the door of wisdom will be opened to you. Then instead of an education, which is very good, you will have wisdom.

The Swami used to say, "We are educated fools with very little wisdom." The whole idea of this esoteric Teaching is to find out, "Who are we? Really, who are we?" We are not R.H. or J.K. We are an ancient soul thousands and thousands of years old, and wisdom comes from knowing who we are and why we are here, what is our purpose, what is our direction. If we can make this a better world for one person, then we have justified our existence, but when we can multiply that by thousands like Tesla, Edison, Ford, and Frank Lloyd Wright, then we are helping the evolution of the planet.

When you have divine dissatisfaction within yourself, then you will seek and you will find. Wisdom is the only thing we can take with us as we pass from house to house of flesh. You can't take mink coats or jewelry or cars or property, but you can take wisdom from lifetime to lifetime to lifetime. It's the most precious thing in the world.

Now if you don't want wisdom, you will remain a cabbage. As Christ said, "Let the dead bury the dead." What did he mean? He was referring to the walking dead. We've seen them. They walk the streets in a complete daze, or they sit looking at television and drinking their beer and there is no joy in living.

205. Very often the search for wisdom begins when people become interested in astrology. Whether you use palmistry or a horoscope or cards or tarot or whatever, it is the beginning of the search and many times it will lead to something else. But if you get stuck on one thing, this is not good, because you may have to stay there this entire lifetime and in the next pick it up and go from there.

In Vedanta they teach that clairvoyance and clairaudience is very charming, but the search for wisdom is the road to God, so don't get stuck on these side roads. These things are fine and useful, but don't make that the goal, the end of wisdom. That's only part of it.

Even if you are lightminded about it, the moment you begin a study of any kind, the door is opened and eventually the study takes over. This is why it is very difficult to do it through spiritualism, because the medium cannot control what is coming in. It may be something good, it may be something bad. This is why they warn you not to fool with it.

Many times fake mediums are playing with power and they don't know what it is, and suddenly they hear or see something and it frightens the hell out of them. This is why many of them become alcoholics or drug addicts. They have opened the door and they can't close it.

206. The Teaching often talks about the philosopher's stone. This means you have attained great wisdom and knowledge and you are actually able to work with alchemy. You begin with the alchemy of the body and as you develop you will find that such things as meat, alcohol, cigarettes, and jealousy, envy and hatred all fall away like unwanted garments. When this happens your whole body chemistry changes.

So the philosopher's stone is a symbol of your having come to that point where you are no longer affected by the things of this world. You are in it but not of it. When you are untouched by the anger, the hatred, the meanness and the ugliness of this world, then you have the philosopher's stone.

207. The Teaching is not exclusive. There are a great many dark forces in the world, and this is a very dangerous Teaching if used in the wrong way. This is the way the Teaching operates: They say, "We send you the people. No one is invited unless they express an interest and this can only happen by one person talking to another."

There will always be dark forces, just as there will always be good and evil. As God is everything, so good and evil must always exist because if everything was perfect we would decay. The height of perfection is decay, with no place to go from there. So we always have these two forces, one operating against the other, in which more good will develop to fight evil and more evil will develop to fight good, and so it keeps on going until one day good will excell over evil.

One day I asked the question, "What is good and what is evil?" The only thing that is evil or bad is to be ignorant and stupid. Wisdom is the thing each person should have. It's the key to your whole life. Wisdom will come through meditation. Reading will help and give you much to guide you, but your real development of wisdom comes through meditation.

We go to school and learn many things but this is not wisdom. Wisdom is discrimination. Wisdom is creativity and wisdom is cultural, and basically that comes through meditation.

Ignorance can be many things. One is provincialism, and to be bigoted, and to be prejudiced, and it only comes with ignorance. Ignorance is the source of evil, but that can be overcome by going out and working with people and getting out of old ruts made with old ideas. Shiva, Shiva, Shiva—the destroyer of the old and the birth of the new, which is tomorrow.

Just as every cell in your body is changing every minute by throwing off old cells and creating new ones, so we should do this with our minds and with our hearts and with all our energies. If we had an idea yesterday and someone can give us a better one tomorrow, throw the old one away and take the new one if it's a better one. But many people will not let go, and this is provincialism. In the East they have this wonderful expression, "Don't convince me with facts, my mind is made up."

208. If you expect something you will receive it. If you don't you won't. As Christ said, "Ask and you shall receive, knock and the door shall be opened unto you." Many people stand at the door but will not knock, because the ego says, who am I to ask? This is false modesty. I like the French word, *demander*. They have no word for ask but *demander* means demand it. This is your birthright and your heritage. You need these things of wisdom and freedom and tolerance and knowledge, but you must ask for them or you'll never have them. You can be a good person and go to church every day in the week, but if you do not ask you will not receive.

At a certain stage of development you have to be extremely careful of what you admire or you'll get it before you realize it. You send out that power of thought and draw it to you. Many times you innocently say, that's very beautiful and it would be nice to have, but you don't really want to be saddled with it as it could become a burden. You must be very careful. This is a law that absolutely works.

209. Light is the opposite of darkness. If you light one match darkness recedes. If you light two, it recedes more. If you light a hundred and a thousand there will be no darkness whatsoever, and the room will be filled with light.

The more Truth and love you put into life, the more darkness recedes. This is why in India Truth is always represented as a diamond: clear cut, perfect in shape, and flawless. There it is, the Light of Truth, like a great diamond sparkling in the sun.

210. Many times when you ask people what they want out of life, they will answer, happiness and security. You can spend your entire life looking for it outside yourself, when all the time it's right there within. Actually, what you're looking for is this special joy of God that's within you. It's there all the time, but you're looking outside for it. When you have this joy you have a special wisdom, and this is what gives you happiness and security.

People talk about security but what is it? Money is not security. Things are not security for they can be taken away just like that. Your house can burn with everything in it and everything is gone. You can be at the top of the ladder of fame and fortune and tomorrow you are nothing, so that is not security. You can be well today and ill tomorrow. Anything can happen, but when you know that wisdom is what you're working with and you know you have that divine wisdom within you, then you are very secure. No matter what comes your way, nobody can take it away from you.

When you can be alone and be delighted with what you are doing and very happy, then you are secure. That's the secret. The majority of people cannot be by themselves. This is the great problem, especially in America where there is this great togetherness. They have to live together, join clubs together, play cards together. When I was in San Francisco, I was invited out to dinner and the people said, "We're going to have a dreadful evening, the television is broken." I said, "Wonderful." They said, "But what will we do?" I said, "We can talk." It was a little awkward at first but we got the thing moving and told jokes and at the end of the evening they said, "We really enjoyed talking this evening. We haven't done this in a long time." This is the thing of joy, to be able to sustain oneself without anything from outside, and when you have that you have everything. Of course, on the other hand, it's not good to go into an ivory tower either.

Psychic Energy

211. Psychic energy is the most perfect form of energy. It comes from the fingertips, the nose, the hands, the mouth, the eyes. Even though man does not know it, that energy is there in his body. This is the energy Dr. Rhine of Duke University has written a book on called *Human Radiations*. It's stronger than ultraviolet rays and it will kill bacteria. It works on both the physical and the subtle bodies, and without it you would die. You generate this energy within you. It comes from the prana in the air and the foods we eat. The more you use the energy the more you have to give. It's an endless supply, so you don't have to stint on it.

Sunlight is an energy of atomic structure and has very beneficial rays, but it's not as fine as psychic energy. Psychic energy has to come from the individual, and the more developed in spirit the individual is, the finer the energy, so that many times they can heal by a thought or a look. This is the highest form of energy there is, and it's opened up not by the individual ego but by being a force for good and the Hierarchy working through you. For instance, imagine yourself as a big pipe through which the energy flows, and when the Hierarchy works through you it becomes that much larger, but when you work through it, it becomes that much smaller. When you tune in on that force it uses you, so it has nothing to do with you personally.

There are several kinds of psychic energy. Materia Lucida is the highest. Fohat is another, and then there is just plain psychic energy. Materia Lucida is the type used in the healing of paralysis. I've seen many miraculous things done with this energy.

This psychic energy is man's link with the universe, with the infinite, and the moment you take away that energy, he becomes ill. People who are ill have no psychic energy. You can keep up that energy by meditation and by not being irritated so that you don't become ill. It takes eight hours to get over the physical reaction from one flare-up of irritation. Irritation, anger and impatience: if you can eliminate these three you can stay on that level of very high energy.

When an individual is ill and in great pain, that energy can be sent by thought and it will actually kill the pain. I just had a call from the parents of a young man who is dying of cancer of the lung. The drugs won't help anymore and he's crawling the walls. He's going to die and there's nothing that can be done, but immediately he got relief from the pain. Anyone can do it.

In healing you absorb the illness of the patient and then throw it off through your aura, so you have to meditate constantly to clear your aura and throw this off or you will come down with one of the illnesses.

When the prana or psychic energy of Earth becomes depleted, the mother ships from other more highly developed planets than ours come down and replace it. And, too, when lightning strikes, it clears the air. You breathe the fresh air after a storm and immediately feel full of energy. It's like taking oxygen. You go outside and breathe four or five times, and you're high on oxygen. This is psychic energy you are inhaling. It makes your body tingle and increases your circulation and makes your blood flow.

On each planet with a higher development than ours, the psychic energy would also be of a higher development, depending on the vibratory rate of that planet. For instance, go back to Atlantis and the pyramids and think about how these things were built by using a magnetic field of thought in which they could move tremendous weights.

We put a limitation on ourselves by thinking we can't do that. It's one of our greatest hang-ups. It's wise to know what you can and can't do, but there is an unlimited force within you and you can do far more than you think you can. You're your own worst enemy.

212. There is an interesting story that explains how psychic energy works. Before one of my disciples sailed for Europe, I told him, "There will be a man on board the ship who is going to be very ill. You will have to get a doctor for him in Paris. This man will be very important to the Teaching one day."

Everything came true just as I had told him. The man developed a blood pressure of 240. My disciple put him into a hospital in Paris and sent for the man's sister who lived in Chicago. She came immediately.

When he could leave the hospital, he and his sister decided to take a place on the Riviera for six months to rest and recuperate. They invited my disciple to go with them. He called me and said, "R., what shall I do?" I said, "If you have the time to go, do so. He needs your energy constantly." They all went to the Riviera and the man who was so ill recovered.

Later his sister came and told me the rest of the story. She said, "We were extremely grateful to your disciple. He took so much of his time and energy to help us. My brother and I enjoyed him so much. He was very amusing and witty and kind, but suddenly my brother became frightened. He said, 'This man has some power over me. I think we should get away.'

'But he's been so kind to us.'

'I feel something emanating from this man. I don't know what it is but I feel he has an influence over me.'

'Well, if you feel that way, we'll go.'

So we packed our bags and my brother left a note telling Mr. S. he could have the villa for as long as he liked because we were going on a trip.

When we got on the train, my brother was the picture of health, but when we were about eighteen or twenty miles away, he began to fade just like a dying flower." She said, "Suddenly he collapsed and died in my arms."

You see, he got out of that ray of psychic energy and he just faded away like an echo. If he had asked what the energy was, he would have been a yogi today and alive and well. He had a very valuable work to do, but it was his choice.

213. As I've told you before, psychic energy is the creative energy that keeps us alive and well. How many people have you known who have retired and lost their incentive for living, the energy drops, they become ill and die?

If you are doing some creative work, you are buoyed up and constantly enthused. This sets fire to your energy and keeps the flame burning, so that if you have an illness or aches and pains you can throw it off by an ecstasy of creativity. In the excitement of it you forget yourself and the negativity leaves. When your negativity keeps piling up and you get into a funk and become discouraged, then you become ill.

This is the basis of healing. The energy of the person being healed is lifted so high that their illness leaves, but you have to forget self. We love to cling to the "I": my pain, my sorrow, my troubles. And to feel sorry for oneself, no matter what the situation, is the very worst thing you can do.

You have eyes to see and ears to hear, and a brain that works somewhat. You have the ability to read all this marvelous literature, and see all the beauties of nature. Look what you have: absolutely everything, but you take it for granted, and when you do this you lose that enthusiasm and love for life, the negative settles in and illness takes over.

Old age is not age of body or mind, but lack of enthusiasm. A dear lady I know in New Mexico is in her nineties and she has more enthusiasm than a fifteen-year-old girl. In her presence you are caught up in it, and it's like a fire on the prairie. You can't resist it. You should try to set young people on fire with ideals and enthusiasm, because this will go with them the rest of their lives.

214. The organ of psychic energy is your appendix. That's the storehouse of your psychic energy. Any creative force is psychic energy. It's like healing—the more energy you give, the more you get.

There is an old Egyptian trick in which you take a glass of water and hold your hand over it and concentrate on what you are doing, and charge that water with your energy for about five minutes and then drink it. And the Rosicrucians recommend that at night you put a glass of water on your bed table so that if you lose your energy at night, the water will act as a conductor and collect it. In the morning you drink it and return your energy to the body.

Animals should not be kept in the sleeping room as they draw psychic energy, and canaries or any caged bird should not be kept as they draw entities. These are all little tricks you can do to conserve your psychic energy.

215. The pine tree and corn have tremendous amounts of psychic energy. Build yourself a pine box. Do not paint it and place your mattress on it. This will give you a bed charged with psychic energy. Pine and corn are loaded with it. It's a special energy from the sun, and these are the only two things on Earth that pick it up. That, and the sap or juices from the pine tree which is made into amber beads. This is also very high in energy, and if you are low in energy

and wear a string of amber beads, this will pick you right up. Speaking of energy, if you wear pearls and your body is unhealthy, they lose their lustre, but when you put them on someone who is healthy they come alive again. Actually, they will eventually die if you put them in a safety deposit box and never wear them.

216. All so-called miracles are performed through psychic energy. Many times when you are sitting looking at an individual the face will blank out, and then as you look, one face after another will appear. I've seen this on a lighted stage where the clothing actually changed as well as the face, and other people in the audience saw it too. Two or three people in the audience with strong psychic energy, or the strong psychic energy of the person on stage would project this phenomenon.

There was a man in Philadelphia by the name of Keely that Madame Blavatsky came to visit in 1887. He had a laboratory and had reversed the law of gravity through levitation. He could make things run on their own just through psychic energy. When he died, everyone called him a fake. They came and tore his laboratory apart looking for pipes or tricks, but there were none, absolutely none. Before his death people came from all over to see him and he would perform these experiments at will, any time, any place. And no one could duplicate them, because he had this thing of psychic energy.

217. One time we experimented with psychic energy and plants out at the Ramakrishna Center in California. They had several bushes that had been transplanted in the wrong season and they were dying, so they asked if we could demonstrate how psychic energy is used in the same way you would use it to heal a sick person. Of the ten shrubs, one died because it was too far gone, but the other nine recovered.

We did another experiment with plants in Glen Cove, Maine one year. There were electrodes connecting the plant with an instrument, and when you would cut or pinch the leaves, the needle on the instrument would register way over on the negative side. Then we would go along and treat the plant with psychic energy, and in less than a minute the plant would be healed, but if we left it alone, it took over an hour and a half for the plant to heal itself.

That's why some people who have a lot of psychic energy can work with these plants, and it's called a green thumb. Some people will cause plants to die when there is disharmony and ugliness, or quarreling and fighting. The planet is affected by this, as we are affected by this. When we talk to plants and flowers and treat them as intelligent beings, they respond to that.

218. Whenever you touch a person, there is an exchange of psychic energy, so you should be careful who you shake hands with. Politicians take this very lightly.

You have all had the experience of being with someone five minutes and you are completely drained of energy. This is a form of vampirism. They sap your energy and throw it away. What you do in this situation is shut it off. Cross your arms, cross your legs and shut them out. This is using discrimination. This is being wise. Don't deplete yourself. Of course, if someone takes your energy who is ill, that's different.

If you receive a letter that is handwritten and you place it in the light in a certain way, you will see the aura of the individual in the handwriting. Useless handwriting is not being discriminating. This is wasted energy.

In Europe when you enter a room you shake hands, and when you leave you shake hands, and if you don't it means you don't like that person; it's an insult. But here in America people rarely shake hands. When you are very close to someone and your auras are in harmony, your physical contact with that person is actually a very important thing. This is why in all the Agni Yoga groups we kiss one another. This is that physical contact that is so important. You benefit by touching someone, and if you touch someone of great quality, you benefit by that. This is why Christ instituted the kissing on the cheek, because in doing this no one can hide their true feelings. If they are insincere, you know immediately. It's like embracing a table leg; nothing happens.

219. Jesus learned how to walk on water from the yogis he studied with in India. In the Teachings they tell you how to practice doing it. It's a sort of do-it-yourself program. You fill the bathtub with water and then you sit on a block of wood. Then you practice to control your breathing from the solar plexis and you have to work at it and work at it, and finally when the piece of wood floats to the surface you know you're doing it.

But it's not good to waste all that energy when you could be putting it into a creative force, or for healing, or in working for peace.

There is a charming story about a young man who studied with the Rishis in India for ten years. They taught him to walk on water, and finally the day came when he called all his family and friends to the side of the lake so he could demonstrate his great achievement. He walked across the lake to the cheers of everyone watching, all except his little brother, who wasn't very impressed. So he said to his brother, "Did you see me walk across on the water?" and the little boy said, "Yes." So he said, "Well, what do you think?" and his brother said, "I can ride across in a boat for ten annas." (Equivalent to 5¢.)

220. Aum is a sacred word and when you utter this in rhythm, in perfect rhythm in a group of people who are in perfect harmony, it becomes a tremendous force of psychic energy. The reason we don't use this more often is that many times there is not enough harmony among the people, and it's not wise to use it unless you are working with a completely open heart. You can use it individually in meditation if you want to.

221. Now, to the question of the dog and cat. People say, "I love my pussy cat. I love my doggie." This is good, and by treating your pet with intelligence and talking to it you will raise its consciousness, but it should never be allowed in the bedroom. They draw in entities and feed on your psychic energy.

You know the old wives' tale about the pussy cat getting onto the chest of the baby and sucking its breath. It isn't that. The pussy cat takes the energy from the baby and the child will die.

In Europe it's a common practice for many of the old grandparents to sleep with the grandchild with the idea of taking the energy of the child, but this is vampirism. It works, but look what they do to the child.

Sometimes a dog will jump up and bite you because they sense this psychic energy around you. Often there is an entity in the dog, and they are frightened of this energy.

In India dogs and pussy cats are not allowed in the temples because the vibrations are too high and the animal could destroy itself. This happened at the Taj Mahal. A dog became so agitated it jumped over the edge and killed itself, and this holds back the development of the animals.

222. I have been asked to explain the difference between psychic gymnastics and physical gymnastics.

Christ said, "Be still and know that I am God." This is that tremendous power that is within each of you to set forth a rhythm. This is a power that you can use, though it's not an action, but an inaction.

For instance, in working for peace you may say, I am only one person, or two or three, or we are fifteen or twenty people praying for peace; and maybe this is not effective, but you don't know. Like the example I gave you before of the man in England, one man alone, a semi-invalid who kept writing letters to the government about the slavery in his country. The day after he died they abolished slavery in England. The potential for good in any individual is unlimited if they are striving and believing. The magic of believing can actually produce results, and this is an inactive activity.

This is hard for the western world to understand, because for them everything has to be on the outside. They look for peace out here when all the time it's inside. It's inside you first of all and then you give it to the other people. It's a quietness within. This is why meditation is good, because you take this quietness into yourself and when you push it out into space, then you are one with the whole of infinity. It's not by rushing out and rushing here and there but by inaction. Hold onto an idea. Don't dissipate it by talking about it. Do it! This is that sacred activity or energy, and it's very important that you preserve it. The outer action is nothing compared to the inner action.

223. In the book, *Letters of Helena Roerich,* it compares the ordinary man and the traveler on the path of Light when it says, "Each blade of grass sets before you a legacy of the forces of nature. Phantoms are for him who sits by the stove, and for you are the waves of luminous matter. Seals and forbiddances are for him who sits in a chicken coop, and for you the creative power of the pure strata of matter."

When you utilize this pure matter the unusual will happen. You set into motion something that is not magic but your natural right to do. It's a natural power like teaching and healing that everyone has a right to use. There is no magic or mystery about it. It's just using, directing and controlling matter to its fullest.

For instance, you can use the power of the matter around a word. You can say, "Stop," or you can explode the words and say *"STOP!"* and in doing this you create a vibratory rate that carries much greater power. So if you can put all words that have a meaning into a powerful use of the word in a sentence, or in its pronunciation, you set up an action by that vibratory rate.

For instance, in swearing if you say, "Damn it," it doesn't mean anything, but if you say, "DAMN IT!" this puts a curse on the thing you're damning and the whole force of the word is made to come alive and vibrate to it. The word itself doesn't mean anything, it's the connotation of the word and how you use it.

224. Manifestations of light are psychic energy. Many times while you are busy working you will see flashes of light, and often at night upon waking suddenly you will see flashes of light before your eyes. When you go to bed and look up at the ceiling you will see myriads of stars. This is a form of psychic energy. In a group of people you often see a ray of iridescent blue light come from the heart and go up to the forehead. It is so brilliant it looks like a neon tube. Many

times a light is around the head, or if you watch the lips of someone who speaks a great truth, a ruby or diamond will fall to the floor. It looks like a jewel but it's light; it's psychic energy.

Fire

225. You asked about fire. White fire is a thing that many times you will see in the atmosphere. You will see flashes of light. Often this indicates that a Mahatma is near by or a truth has been spoken. When an individual will say, I have seen a Mahatma or the Mahatmas said this or that, over their head you will see this white fire which verifies it, so that you're not working by guesswork or by wishful thinking. If a Mahatma appears, They tell you, "Challenge it," and right over the head will appear this fire.

Now it doesn't matter what color it is because darkness can never produce light. The blue fire is often used in healing. And many times people who are approaching discipleship will see this blue fire. It is given to them as a proof.

I'll tell you the story of J.H. After the first night he came to class J. went home and to bed, and as he pulled the covers up they burst into flames. He started to put them out and then he realized this was not a "fire" fire but a spiritual fire. It looked like a "fire" fire, only it was blue and it didn't burn. This happens frequently.

Very often this is a great creative fire. In this case, J.H. had a job to do. He was to build power stations all around the world that would draw energy from the universe. He came to me and said, "Is this what I am supposed to do?" And I said, "Yes." We were given a special book for him to read; *The Prodigal Genius*—the story of Tesla's life.

Unfortunately, he didn't come through with the assignment. As They say, the time is now to do these things for the benefit of the world, but if we don't do them, there is no blame. The job will be given to someone else and it will only be delayed a few years.

Some years ago I knew an artist who had lived with the Indians in British Columbia for two years. They allowed him to photograph this blue fire. They would begin by beating their drums and clapping their hands and chanting and dancing around a physical fire in this big room made of twigs and clay. It was like a large hogan which they used for religious purposes and healing. They would start with slow movements and build up and up, and about an hour after they started the ceremony a ring of blue fire about two and a half feet high would appear around the room. About two hours after that the fire had reached all the way up to the ceiling. This is spiritual fire. The Indians can do this because they live very close to the cosmic laws. They obey these laws.

In Taos when the Indians are going to kill a deer, they have a special meeting the night before in which they explain to the deer that they must kill him for food and will not kill any more than they need. It's the same with the rabbits. They explain they must have food for their women and children, and they ask forgiveness for this and never kill in excess. People laugh at them, but they know the law and obey it.

This is why in Taos we had so many miraculous healings. The chief had cancer for twenty-two years and overnight he was well again. His wife had been blind for years and in fifteen minutes she had her vision restored. These people have a great purity. They live so close to the letter of the word of God, and have such pure ethics, they're unlimited. They don't think it can't be done and so spectacular things happen.

226. What is Fohat? It's a kind of cosmic electricity; a higher form of psychic energy. Thought is the highest manifestation of this energy. Sometimes when you are talking to an individual, a blue flame goes right from the top of his head up to the ceiling. This is a demonstration of this electricity. It will not burn. It's a manifestation of the light of illumination. It usually occurs in a room where we are all sitting and talking. Suddenly, there will be a great burst of light or a glow will appear in different colors. It helps if you are clairvoyant. No, this is not the aura. This is a separate thing. This is Fohat. Sometimes there will be a great fire in the corner of the room or in back of an individual. It will be blue or white, like a forked tongue of fire. Many people, when they see this, start putting it out, and then they realize it's not a fire that burns.

In Tibet on New Year's day, which is February 15th or 18th, the fire flowers burst forth. The idea of the snow maiden comes from these fires which suddenly burst forth on the top of the highest mountains, and burn for about twenty-four hours. This is psychic energy. Roerich did a series of paintings called *Fire Flowers.*

The burning bush of Moses is also a manifestation of this energy.

And when you hear of the eternal light that burns in tombs, this is the same thing. When they broke open the Rosencrans tomb, there was this light. Manly Palmer Hall has done a book in which he tells about all these eternal lights. They are found in South America, in Indian caves, in Greece and various other places around the world. This is the fiery energy that is Agni.

227. The Teaching talks a great deal about creative fire. This happens when you can create a fire within another individual's heart, when you can set them on fire. It's something that does not exist in the physical or the Subtle World, but is manifested through your fire igniting theirs. Again, this is unity. It's an invisible thing that happens between two people, and it can only happen when that individual is caught up, inspired and transcended. It's an experience that's very difficult to describe. It's more than enthusiasm, it's an actual fire of the spirit.

When the Tashi Lama comes into a temple, all the candles light up by his presence. Both my Guru and his wife, Madame Roerich, saw this happen over and over. This is His fire of psychic energy. It's called the fire of Agni. This is why Agni is one of the most ancient fires.

If you ignite this fire within another person and they become aflame with the Teaching, that flame will exist forever and ever, from lifetime to lifetime. It's like being struck by lightning and nothing, but nothing can turn you off.

You see, the intellect is the great stumbling block because it wants to say, "Could this be true?—well, I doubt it." And the moment you doubt the door is closed for that whole lifetime.

Sometimes a spectacular healing will bring about a great love for the Teaching, but after six months or so, they will say, well, maybe it was this or that, and they lose it. What they try to do is discredit it and bring it down to their level.

People always try to tear things down to their level. It's like the old saying, "God made man in His image and then man turned around and made God in his." It's a natural law of the Earth people. If you cannot look up into the heavens and see the stars, then you say there are no stars. Christ said, "There are none so blind as those who will not see, nor so deaf as those who will not hear." When you explain something in the Teaching to these people and they say, "I do not understand," it means, "I do not want to understand." When you hear them say this, it tells you the whole story. Walk off and leave them, because you're wasting their time and yours. They won't accept it.

228. I have explained to you before how at the time of the final initiation you are taken above ten thousand feet and taught to handle the fires of space, and how when you are healing and go beyond a certain point you cannot stop or you will be burned to ash.

You have read of these odd cases about people who are sitting in a chair and every part of the person is burned, so that not even the bones are left and the chair is not even scorched. This is that fiery energy. They have too much psychic energy, or they have tuned in to this high psychic energy in some way and are dissolved, burned by that invisible fire. In some way they have come in with it, but are not using it. It may be they have developed a very high consciousness, but have no direction and don't know what they're doing, and suddenly it builds up to a point where it burns them to ash.

They will probably come back very quickly and next time they will do something with it. Many times, for instance, a man or woman who has a good heart by being benevolent and kind and good will open the heart center and have a heart attack, or they may open the lung center and have consumption, or they may open the chakra on the top of the head or the eye of dharma and it affects them like a brain tumor. This is why it's very wise to have instruction.

229. When the Teaching speaks of the Fiery Heart, this is the heart center, not the physical heart.

Again you go back to the Catholic religion. They have this heart of Christ and the fire with the two flames; one is physical and one is spiritual, and it's a combination of the two that creates the opening of the heart.

And with that open heart you can fire another heart into a creative thing of enthusiasm. Enthusiasm is like fire in a dry field.

Of course there is also your black fire. Hitler is an example of black fire. He was a black magician. In *Psychic Discoveries Behind the Iron Curtain,* they mention that his teacher was a great white yogi, but the student turned it around and used it for his own purpose. Many of his speeches wouldn't even make sense. He would stand up and just make noises and the people were captured by this fire of power and evil and it spread throughout the crowds. It didn't matter whether they understood him or not, they cheered wildly because he was able to fire them.

Of course, if you are able to do this constructively, then this is beautiful. Actually this is what the theater is used for. Asvaghosha is the patron saint of the theater. He was a great Tibetan Guru. He taught his disciples and they would do these plays in the market place. They traveled all over India from town to town. The theater is basically a thing of metaphysics in which the individual can be taught a lesson through entertainment.

Even today many actors and actresses do a meditation before a performance to lift the consciousness of the audience and heal any person in the theater. For instance, *The Cocktail Party* (by T. S. Eliot) is a complete occult play. Somerset Maugham, too, was a great occultist. He had a guru in India. This is how They work with the message. The Teaching has been spread in this way for hundreds of years, all down through history. It's not just a thing of today. The trouble is, people see not and they hear not.

230. Individuals who are filled with peace, harmony and love attract others to them from that heart element, like a moth to the flame, and this is what is called "beyond the boundaries of karma." For instance, the people who come into the Teaching come through some form of motivation, such as a healing, or a desire for consciousness, or for wisdom, or to be a better person, but that motivation is the thing that is beyond karma because you do it yourself.

Some people can just walk into a hospital room, and even though they say nothing the patient feels better. Many doctors have this quality; call it enthusiasm or whatever you like, it is a quality that reaches out and touches the individual. Like this cancer case I was on up in Canada. The patient was told to go home and die, and naturally he was completely discouraged. But the moment his confidence was restored he changed his attitude, got out of bed, put on his clothes and went out.

Of course, you can never tell a person they are going to die. This is a terrible thing to do. It may look like they are dying but you never can tell. My uncle was a physician, and he told my family when I was sixteen that if I lived to be seventeen it would be a miracle. He's dead and I'm still alive. There is always hope if we can reach out and hold on to it. That hope is the fire they speak about, and it attracts like a moth to the flame. And with it you can move mountains.

If we are motivated by that fire and if we strive, we will accomplish whatever we set out to do in spite of ourselves. We make our own stumbling blocks, and we say this or that is impossible. Nothing is impossible if we really want to do it, but you really have to want to do it and you can't sit down and twiddle your thumbs and hope it will happen. You really have to work at it. This is the creative fire. Again this is what Agni means, that fire of enthusiasm.

Often I tell young people who are going into painting or music, you may not be a genius, not all people are, but you may have a fine sense of color and develop into a great painter. You should never discourage a painter or musician by saying you can never do that. Instead, light a spark of enthusiasm or daring within them and they may go right to the top. They have to be fired with a burning enthusiasm, and that can only come through the heart. Two examples are Tesla, who had that burning enthusiasm to bring all those inventions to the world, and Frank Lloyd Wright; and both men had this burning desire to accomplish their life's work, and nothing but nothing was going to stop them.

231. The fiery purification and special fire they speak of in the Teaching would be earthquakes, tidal waves and fiery things of this sort. Occasionally, when the consciousness of mankind does not

move along as it should, these things take place. They are caused by the thinking and the actions of man himself. This is a cosmic law. It's actually not a destructive thing when an earthquake hits or a volcano explodes. It's a clearing up of the old garbage, and what you do is get rid of the deadwood, and the people who are caught in it will move on to a higher evolution and come back again. If humanity won't move any other way, They'll burn the schoolhouse down.

Enthusiasm

232. The festival of the spirit is enthusiasm. All people should develop enthusiasm, because when the fire has gone out the enthusiasm has gone and you're walking around like a dead duck.

The killing of enthusiasm is a very, very bad thing. Many times a person will have an idea and they are very enthusiastic about it, and then someone will say, "Oh, that's been done before," or "Well, I don't know, I don't think that's such a good idea." When this happens, look out; this is the sign of a dark force. They kill enthusiasm wherever possible, and when enthusiasm is killed, many times the creative ability of that individual will die. It's stifled and killed.

If something is original even though it's not perfect, it will still have some good quality. Point out that quality. I once heard a lecture by Mr. Tiffany. He was talking to a group of artists, and he showed us a very large flashy diamond ring and another diamond that was rather small. He talked about quality. At first, you were attracted by the large stone, but when he talked about the cut and purity of the smaller stone, the large one actually began to look cheap and brassy. Apply this idea to enthusiasm. If there is quality in the creative ability, say, "Well, it may not be a Michaelangelo, but you have beautiful color or beautiful lines." Don't be phony, but you can always find one good thing to be enthusiastic about.

For instance, a man came to me in New York who was working in advertising. He said, "R., I'm writing copy on a car that's no good. I think it's a pile of junk, but I need the money. I have to support my family. What shall I do?"

I said, "Don't misrepresent the car, but there must be something good about it." He said, "Yes, the brakes are good." "Then take that theme," I told him, "and tell people how valuable good brakes can be and how they may save your life."

He built the entire advertising campaign on that one feature, and it was very successful.

When you find something to be enthusiastic about, don't keep it a state secret. For instance, when you go into a restaurant and are served good food, tell someone about it. Tell the waitress, the manager or the cashier. Say, "This is wonderful coffee." They will probably look at you and say, "What?" because they expect a complaint, not a compliment. Usually when food or service is good, people say nothing, but if it's bad they really raise a fuss.

One day we were on a trip and stopped at a restaurant for lunch. The waitress had three or four difficult customers, and they were giving her a very bad time. Then someone said something pleasant to her and she smiled. She had the most beautiful smile—like the sunshine.

When she came to our table, I said, "My dear, you have given me great pleasure just to see your smile. It's wonderful. It's beautiful."

From that moment on she smiled at everyone. Tell people when they have done a good job. This encourages them to do even better. Everyone needs encouragement, everyone! If just one person believes in you completely, you can accomplish miracles.

Drugs

233. There are no short cuts to God Consciousness. That's why drugs like LSD are of no value whatsoever because it's a short cut. Many times they have very bad effects on the individual. If the consciousness is not high enough to take it, it can destroy you.

What a terrible karma Aldous Huxley has for publishing this information about drugs in a book for all these people to read. All Teachings say if you are a writer and you write misinformation, you are karmically responsible for every reader who reads what you have written. If you write a story about murder and someone reads it and goes out and commits a murder because of this influence, the karma is on you, the writer. Even if the book on murder is stated to be fiction and a weak mind reads it, you are responsible for all your readers. This is an esoteric law.

234. Imperil creates rheumatism and arthritis. Drugs also create rheumatism and arthritis. More than that, drugs and alcohol destroy

the spiritual consciousness for the next life. I've had cancer patients who were climbing the wall in pain and who wouldn't take drugs to relieve the pain, but they got relief from psychic energy. When people take drugs for great pain it affects their next life, but not in the astral.

Addicts are affected because they die faster, and then they must remain in the lower astral until their life span is fulfilled and they are released to go on. While they are in the astral they attach themselves to other people for gratification of their habit. Alcoholics, too, gravitate to bars, even the most elegant ones, where they can be gratified.

Recently this young musician called me and said he had taken LSD about a year and a half ago, and now when he wakes up in the morning he is completely withdrawn and can't get back into the world. The drug experience keeps recurring. I told him to stop meditating immediately. You should never meditate for two years after having taken acid. It takes that length of time to get it out of your system.

235. In Manly Palmer Hall's big book, it was Pythagoras who was interested in form and the relationship between mathematics and forms.

Aldous Huxley also did a book called *The Disappearance* in which he describes how they built a vehicle made of mirrors with twelve sides, and when a person stepped inside he would disappear into another dimension. This is part of the form they were talking about. Huxley was a Vedantist and mystic, and very well trained, so evidently he knew.

He also discovered peyote from the Indians, and then he wrote a book on it; and actually this was a terrible thing for him to do, because he is karmically responsible one thousandfold for every reader. But this was sensational and he got carried away with it.

The Indians use peyote for the purpose of being clairvoyant. I worked very closely with the Indians in Taos. One part of the pueblo would not touch it, and another part of the pueblo would use it, but only for special religious things. They showed me the plant and blossoms and everything, and they asked me to sit in and see psychically what was happening, but we never could get together. They only use it twice a year for a religious experience. These people are very mystical.

Of course the best thing is meditation, because the moment you get into the use of drugs you get into the lower astral and you cannot go into the Fiery World. The only way you can do that is by meditation.

Auras

236. The aura is the energy of the consciousness. It's like a glove, like the hand would be the body and the glove the aura, and at death the glove is taken off and it floats in space until it dissolves. The body is nothing but an old overcoat and it's thrown away.

And as the double of this body disintegrates, then you can come back for reincarnation, but if the muscles are built up, then it takes that much longer for the body to disintegrate and that much longer to come back.

The aura around your head changes color with your thinking, but the aura around your body remains more or less the same. Green auras are intellect. Blue are spiritual. Green and blue are harmonious. Red is the color of excitement. Blue-red is the color of love. Orange-red is the color of violence. An acid orange means frustration and the heat of passion. Yellow is healing and stimulates thought and striving.

For instance, your healers have a golden yellow aura and around that is a touch of purple, which is the color of Hierarchy. In the Teaching they say, the fastest way to God consciousness is through healing because you take away pain and sorrow. That is why the aura is always touched with the color of Hierarchy.

If the person is talking through the intellect, the aura will turn a brilliant green. If what they are saying is from the spirit, it will be all blue.

Usually in your early meditations you begin to see blobs of color. This is very, very good. The first color you see is usually a blob of a brilliant luminous blue and then you see lavenders and purples and reds, etc. Many times in a room there will be swimming lights of color. This is psychic energy.

The intensity of the color of the aura is greatest in a state of repose or sleep, or when you are completely involved and creating.

When you are in that state between sleep and awaking, you are most clairvoyant, or when you are doing some very highly creative work and are under a great deal of tension, this is when your clairvoyance is wide open. Your clairaudience is open then, too.

237. Meditation prevents the subtle body from becoming damaged. The aura is the protective net, and many times if people are

sending you ugly thoughts they will try to penetrate your aura, and then you have to meditate and throw that off.

You do the same thing when you are treating ill people. Every once in awhile you have to clear your aura through meditation or you will take on their illness.

238. Dark spots in the aura can indicate illness or chaotic conditions around the individual, but you must be able to distinguish which it is. If it is illness, a little tail will come down to the affected part. For instance, if there is a heart condition the little tail will come right down and point to the heart. A dark spot in the aura without the tail could be chaotic conditions within the individual himself or around him, like friends or family or someone in the immediate vicinity. If you see this you should tell him because it might be an impending accident.

But, if you see illness in the aura you may not tell the person unless he asks. You are not to play God. Always remember this. However, if you are in a restaurant and a waiter or waitress comes up to you and says, "Oh, my God, I'm going mad with this pain," and if you know what to do, offer help at once. This is the Lord speaking to you, but if they say nothing, you too must remain silent.

One day I was in my favorite little Italian restaurant; it's so wonderful, I love it. The waitress came up and said, "Oh, my tooth is driving me crazy." So I asked, "Do you want some relief for it?" She said, "Oh, anything." I said, "Bring me a plate, some matches, a piece of brown paper, a few pins and a pair of scissors." We put the plate down and made a funnel of the brown paper. You roll the paper very tightly and pin it, like a wigwam. (This is an old, old remedy I learned from a French farmer.) Cut a small hole in the top and set the paper on fire. Remember it must be brown paper. As this burns you balance it with a knife so it doesn't fall and start a fire. The burned ash will stain the plate with a greenish, yellowish substance. Pick this up with the end of your finger and put it directly on the tooth, and it will stop any toothache immediately. I told her, "Go to your dentist tomorrow, but this will give you relief tonight."

If you see a person in a great deal of pain but they have not asked you for help, you may pray for them that, if it is their karma, then relieve this pain. That you can do, but otherwise you must not interfere.

Healing

239. The question was asked, "What is an imponderable substance transmuted to imponderable energy?"

An example of this is the idea of thought used in healing through absent treatment. This is done by people working through the occult; Christian Science also uses the same principle. This energy is transmitted by the eye, the hands and the mouth, as well.

Now in absent treatment, all you have to have is the name of the person, their age, the birth month, the year and day they were born, and where they are now, and with this information you can send the thought like an arrow. As I have told you before, in the East the arrow is always referred to as thought going directly to the individual. There may be two or three people by the same name, so this is why we ask for the date of birth or, if they are married, what was their name at birth.

Actually, on Tuesday night, which is healing night, there are long lists of individuals that we work with. We don't recite the names because it would take two or three hours to do it, but collectively these names have asked for that help and they get it.

There is no fee and no acceptance of any gifts. What the individual must do when they are healed is help twenty or thirty other people. It is very important that you do not heal anybody unless they ask for it and agree to help twenty or thirty other people in repayment.

Any service done in the Lord's name, whether it is volunteer work at a hospital or in a library, or taking soup to a neighbor who is ill, or helping anyone in any way is payment. Many times people get fouled up in this because they want to help someone and they say I will take on the debt. Don't let them do it. We all have enough karma without taking on somebody else's. Then you get another stock answer, "Oh, we help people all the time." When you hear that, look out.

Never put someone on a healing list unless they request it, because you're interfering with the karma of that individual. Many times someone you love very much is very ill, and you must have a great sympathy for them and you want to help, but you must keep hands off. You may pray for them, but it is not good to do a (healing) meditation for someone unless they ask for it. This is a very fine point in yoga. Group prayer, yes, but don't meditate for them because what you are doing is opening a door for them that they may not be ready for and may not want.

240. In Marion, South Dakota there is a group of healers called the Tieszen Group, founded by old Peter Tieszen. (Tieszen Clinic, P.O. Box 248, Marion, S.D. 605-648-3761.) They are Dutch, but were driven out of Holland a long time ago. They went to Russia and were driven out by persecution and then they came to America. They are bone healers, the only bone healers (in the Western world) I have ever heard of.

One of my disciples had a broken arm when he was fourteen, and it was set and healed crooked. His mother took him to the Tieszen Clinic and the doctor said, "This is going to hurt for a few minutes," and he broke the arm over again and then just made two or three passes over the arms and said, "Don't play baseball for a couple of days." The arm was absolutely healed. My contact with them has been through their sending me cataract cases to heal. Apparently this is something they can't heal.

Old Peter used to have a farm but now he has a clinic. They work on cases of broken backs and vertebra. The President of Morton Salt went there with a very bad case of palsy that he'd had for thirty years. Now, as you know, palsy can't be healed medically, but they healed him. Very gratefully he wrote out a check for ten thousand dollars, but they said, "No, your bill is $2.00 a day for your room and fifty cents for the interview with the doctor." They are obviously not trying to make money from this. "But," they said, "there is a poor woman who lives down the road who just lost her husband, and she is about to lose her farm because she can't pay the mortgage. If you want to do something, help her." So he went down and bought machinery and hired a couple of men, and made her farm a paying business.

Each of old Peter's grandsons was given the title of Doctor. At one time the AMA was going to close them down, but thousands of people rose up and testified as to what they had done for them and how they had been healed, so the State passed a special law allowing these people to practice and use the degree of Doctor. They have no nurses, so if you go there you must take a relative or friend along. The food is good, but plain, and served in a cafeteria.

One of the most dramatic stories I've ever heard was of a young man who had broken his leg and gangrene had set in. He was taken to the clinic and they removed a section of bone from the leg. He lay flat in bed, and at the end of three months they took an x-ray. There was a milky substance in the place where the bone had been. At the end of six months the x-ray showed that area to be a little more solid, and at the end of nine months the bone had grown as one and his leg was perfect. Now, medically they say you can't grow a bone.

Bone healing is an extremely rare form of healing. In the East the only place it can be done is in Tibet.

There's an interesting story of how a group of high Lamas actually grew a hand that had been bitten off by a mountain lion. First a stub of a hand grew back, and then the fingers. In a matter of nine hours it had grown back. These men had stopped the caravan when the lion bit off the hand and they sat around the man and concentrated on this and someone photographed it as it was happening. It was grown back into the pattern of the astral hand which was still there.

The growing of this hand happened to a very high Lama and the growing was done by a group of very high Lamas. It did not happen to an ordinary person, but this soul was very pure with no unbelief.

What you do in healing is treat the pattern of the astral body. The same is true with shock treatments for the mentally disturbed. In this case the astral body is slightly out and what you do is put it back in. After the shock treatment the patient is always a little fuzzy, and this is caused by the astral body being a little to one side.

Rudolph Steiner has a school in Switzerland in which they work with abnormal children, and what they do is work with the astral body to get it back into the physical, and they do wonderful, wonderful work. They are a metaphysical group and the only group that works in this way.

There are cosmic laws and your esoteric groups work with them instead of against them. I'm not saying that the medical doctors are no good. They are good, but if they were occult doctors they would be excellent, because they could look at the patient and tell what was wrong instead of guessing or trying this or that treatment. The doctor who works only on the physical and ignores the astral is aware of only half the problem, whereas the doctor who works on the astral body knows this reflects on the physical. In the Teaching They say, "We are very interested in doctors."

We had a very wonderful thing happen to a friend of Dr. G.'s. Dr. R. was one of the finest bone surgeons in America, a man of about forty-five at the height of his profession, and suddenly all the nerves in his arm broke and he couldn't move it. Being a doctor, he knew nothing could be done for this, so he called Dr. G. and said, "Look, can you get this yogi friend of yours to come over and work on this? I need my left arm. I'm too young to have this happen." He couldn't even hold a book or a cigarette, so we went to work on him and in two months all the feeling in his arm came back. Now this man said, "I'm going to take this and apply it to my patients, because this is a whole new approach to healing that I can bring to them."

This is a very wonderful doctor and a fine man, but even so this is a pretty broad thing for him to accept. In this case he could be helped because it was not the loss of bone, just nerves. Up to now, when the body began to disintegrate it couldn't be rebuilt again, at least not in America. Only recently there have been heart transplants and kidney transplants being done in America because the people are saying it can be done.

There's another interesting story on this thing of healing. One of my students in New York was working for General Electric. They had built this special machine to treat arthritis, but it wasn't very successful; however, there was one doctor in Detroit, a little bit of a man, a chiropractor who was tremendously successful and he had reams of patients who were healed. "So," my student told me, "they sent me out to see why this man had such great success and the others didn't. The doctor was nice and cooperative and I said, 'Would you let me see how you operate this machine?' and he said, 'Of course,' and called a patient in and turned some knobs and some lights came on, and I kept waiting for him to turn the machine on but he never did. It was warmed up and that's all. He never pushed the *on* button." This man was a healer and didn't know it.

While we are on the subject of healing, there is the story of this man who went to Lourdes in France for a healing. He was terribly, terribly ill, and as he prayed for a healing he saw this child who was very crippled, and so he changed his prayer and said, "Oh Lord, heal this child. Let me go but give the healing to the child," and with that prayer he had an instant healing. He had transcended beyond his own desires and his unselfish thought is what did it. The minute you can get the ego away from the individual anything can happen. Because of his love and pity and compassion for the child he was healed.

The child was not healed because karmically it had not earned the healing, and probably he would not have been healed either if his thoughts had been only for himself. Sacrifice is the fastest way we can develop. When we can think of others instead of ourselves, then we can really move.

241. The deodar is a fascinating tree and often used in healing. It grows in Texas and California. Deodar is a Sanskrit word meaning "Gift of God," and in the East is called an electric machine.

You kick off your shoes and take a branch in each hand and do some deep breathing for about ten minutes, and you will pull in the magnetic field of the tree and also the solar ray. It's the same reaction as throwing a pine bough onto an open fire, and it goes pssst and explodes. The pine tree is very high in energy and this is released. This is atomic energy. Corn also has this energy. The pine and the corn both get their energy directly from the sun and the magnetic force of the Earth.

I worked with this case of a beautiful young girl who came out to California on a stretcher plane. She had cancer of the hip and the doctors in New York wanted to amputate. She called me as a last resort. I said, "You are in such bad shape and I don't know how far the cancer has progressed inside, but if you want to come I will do what I can."

She had no energy. She had to be carried. So I drove her out to the park where there was a large grove of deodar trees. The first day I carried her. The second day she walked with assistance, with my arm around her. The third day she walked alone and in two weeks she went home well.

What happens in cancer cases is that your energy goes and the disease takes over. Around every cell there is an electrostatic field and each cell links to the other cells, and when this field dies and the cells can't do their work—can't be born fast enough to rejuvinate the body—the cell goes wild and tears tissue. If you can replace the energy, you can control the disease. It's that simple.

In India and Tibet where there is no cancer, they have been taking these simple precautions for hundreds of years. They eat no meat, only lamb and fish and foul, because the fear of the animal when it is killed creates imperil, which is like a crystal, and these crystalline deposits form at the nerve endings, cutting off the energy.

This is why Tibetan musk is very good for cancer, or any pine tree, because it is pure energy. Tibetan musk is found high up in the Himalayas, above 18,000 feet, where a pink meteoric dust falls on the snows. The dust then penetrates the snow and feeds a musk plant under the snow. The deer are attracted by this odor and dig down under the snow to find this plant. When they eat it, the musk enters their glands. Then they continue to smell this musk odor and they go mad trying to find where it's coming from, and consequently throw themselves over the cliff and die. The Lamas go and cut out the glands and this is dried and carefully preserved. It's extremely expensive and hard to come by. Musk runs about three to five thousand dollars a pound. There are substitutes, but the way to tell if you have real musk is to have five people join hands and the first person holds the vial of musk in his closed hand and the fifth person at the other end will feel the energy of the musk. It's absolutely fool proof.

Tibetan musk is the highest form of psychic energy because it goes back to the meteoric dust from the other planets. This is not a cure-all but it is very good for balancing the entire body and to help the consciousness. It comes in little tiny pellets and it's advised to take no more than two small grains a day. It is not a drug. You cannot take large doses in the hope of expanding your consciousness. It won't work. It's to give you energy because as long as your energy is high you cannot become ill, but it's when your energy is low that disease and illness take over. This is why it's very good to know about musk and deodar and such things.

Another cause of depletion of energy is anger and hatred and criticism and negativity. Medically it has been proven that if someone steps on your toe and you flare up in anger, it takes eight hours for your body to expel the effects. Imagine what you are doing to yourself if you are angry for a week. When people say, "You're breaking out in a rash of gossip," or "What's eating you," these are manifestations of your thinking. Anxieties are bad, because you attract to yourself whatever it is you are thinking. If you have a negative thought, say, "Get out, I haven't time for you." You are captain of your ship, so run it and don't allow a mutiny.

In healing you can command a fever to go down by counting to ten. You see, the body is a part of divine intelligence and will obey you, but we let it run wild and don't command it to obey us. If you have a pain, order it out. Just say, "Get out," and it will go.

By the same token, whatever you think about you will bring to yourself. If you think of sickness, you will draw it to you. If you think negative, you become negative. If you think positive, you become positive.

One day in New York, J.D. was at my apartment and his uncle called and wanted him to go to lunch, and J. didn't want to go so he said, "Oh, I'd love to go but I'm too ill. . ." I said, "Don't say that." Within a half hour he was so ill he had to go to bed. This sort of thing works faster on those who are working with Truth because they should know better.

242. If a dog is barking and making a great noise and you want to meditate, send a mental message to the dog to be quiet, and do you know it will quiet down? Thought is a very powerful thing. It is actually more powerful than words because so many people resist what you say, but a thought can penetrate where a word won't.

For instance, absentee healing is much more effective than contact healing because the individual being healed usually has a lot of fixed ideas about how it's going to operate or how they are going to work with it. But absentee healing is a constructive thing and you send thought for the benefit of that particular person and his ego doesn't resist. He won't build up a wall of resistance; consequently he is much more open and the healing is much more successful.

Contact healing is psychologically important to the patient. Many times he will say, "I can't see anything or feel anything." It's like two glasses of water. In one you put salt, and then you move them around and you say, "Which one has two elements in it and which one has one?" It's the same with healing. You can't see it or feel it, but the result is the patient gets well.

People will say, "You're not taking my temperature or my pulse, so how can it work?" It's when a constructive thought dominates a negative thought. When negative thoughts develop in you and you can't let go of them, then they develop into illness. If you can hold onto constructive thinking and sustain this attitude and bring it up to a high level, you will never become ill. Actually, healing is lifting the consciousness up to a very, very high level, and in that moment the ego leaves and "boom," you're healed. But as long as the ego is involved, the illness will not go.

243. In the book, *Fiery World,* it says, "The fiery eye projects the ray of light if it focuses its attention upon a significant object." This is magnetic and follows the laws of the common magnet. This refers to the ability to heal with the eyes. Roerich had the ability to heal with the eyes. Instead of treating with the hands you treat with the eyes.

I must warn you: be very, very careful in doing this because I've ruined my eyesight by being careless and over-did it, and it brought on all my eye trouble. When you do this too much you damage the eyesight because what you do is use the fire right through the eye to heal. It's very beneficial and very good, but you must be careful not to do too much of this kind of healing.

In the Teaching they speak of killing the mad dog with the eye of the yogi. In the Eastern countries like India it can be done but not here in America. You can imagine what would happen! The people here are not ready for it.

There is also an exchange of energy from art objects or artifacts, because whatever the artist puts into the painting the viewer receives.

244. Materia Lucida is psychic energy and is found in all matter. Nikola Tesla was the first person to say that around all matter was energy and the scientific world laughed at him. Then Einstein came along and proved him right.

Dr. Rhine of Duke University has done a whole book on the radiations of psychic energy. This is how healing is done: by utilizing this psychic energy you direct your energy to another individual and raise the level of their energy. If there is illness or disease, it leaves.

As you all know, if the energy is depleted then illness takes over, but a revitalization of that psychic energy can cause an instant healing.

Around each cell is a tiny electrostatic field of energy, and when all these cells are connected to one another this creates a great battery in the human body and gives us a sense of well being. But when these cells are not functioning as they should, as when cancer sets in, then the electrostatic field around each cell dies, the cell goes wild and tears the tissue. When you heal cancer you revitalize the electrostatic field around the cell and thus bring the cell back to its normal function. This is why many times a hopeless case of cancer can have an instant healing.

One of my disciples had cancer of the breast and was very upset about this and overnight she had a complete healing. It wasn't a matter of faith, because I've seen people cured who had no faith whatsoever. It's also a thing of karma. They have earned this in some past life.

Healing is a very scientific operation. The psychic energy is first applied to the psychic or astral body and that reflects on the physical body. Medicine only works on the physical body. They ignore the subtle body, and that's the most important part.

During World War II we had a young man come to us who had lost his arm and shoulder. He said they did everything they could to save the arm, but it was either remove the arm and shoulder or he would die. He complained that over the three-year period since this happened, he continued to have phantom pains in this shoulder. He had an artificial arm but the astral body was still suffering from this injury. So we went to work on the astral body and the pain went away completely. He then brought about twenty-eight veterans who were suffering from astral pains in various parts of their bodies where they had had operations and they all got results.

Mental illness is a breakdown of cells in the brain. Many times this is caused by people becoming discouraged or depressed, and they become lost.

In our prayer we say, "May we be a light for those who have lost the way," and that's what we mean. When we say, "May we be a bridge, a boat, for those who wish to go to the other side," this means the spiritual consciousness. We are like a boatman crossing the river of Santana or stream of spiritual life, and we are offering to bring people to the other side.

245. You must never impose a healing on another individual. We may love them very much, but if they do not ask for it or take the responsibility for it, you must not do it. If you do, you are interfering with the free will of that person. You may cure the disease and if they are not aware of their debt to the Lord, you make them irresponsible. You have interfered with their karma.

You can pray for them and you may ask if you can help take away the pain, if you see they are in pain. Often you may wish you could take their pain upon yourself, but you must not do it.

In healing you are using the highest form of psychic energy, and if the individual is not aware of his debt to the Lord for this, you are dragging this energy down into the dust. This is what Christ meant when he said, "Touch me not." They were not ready to take this energy and use it wisely and be grateful for it.

We must never interfere with another individual. Even with disciples we can only suggest. Man has absolute free will and we cannot play God. If someone wants help, they will ask for it and then you will give it. If they do not know about psychic healing, this is their karma. They have not earned the right to know, and you must not interfere with karma.

If someone is having a heart attack or something like that and you are the only person there, it is your duty to do all you can to help, but not a healing unless they ask for it.

246. Often people come to me and say, "How can I be of service?" One of the greatest ways to serve humanity is through healing. To illustrate this, I was talking to one of my disciples on the phone one day. He knew I had just come back from a bad cancer case in Canada. He said, "Can we help?" and I said, "Of course. The more people who work together on a thing like that the better, because you condense the energy and focus it." He said, "Why didn't you tell me that?" and I said, "Because I simply can't." If we have to give orders to people, this is no good. This is the thing of free will and I must not impose my will in any way, shape, or form, even to a disciple. If they come to me and say, "I give you permission to direct me in any way you see fit," then I can, but otherwise, I would be violating a cosmic law by telling you to do something. You have free will and no one has the right to impose their will on you. Only if you offer, then all is fine and good.

When you say to the Hierarchy, "Use me as you will," They will, but unless you say "Use me," They won't because that would be a violation of free will.

If you impose your will over someone else, that may be the worst thing in the world for them. You may be pushing them into something they will resent later on and that's no good. It has to be absolutely free. All wars, all difficulties in families have been caused by imposing the will of one person over another. The Hierarchy is against that.

247. Oftentimes when people have had a healing, they give credit to the pills they took instead of to the Lord. All they have to

say is, "I have had a healing of the Lord," but what they are trying to do is gyp the Lord. When this happens they incur much karma. What has happened is a sacred thing, and what they are doing is tearing it down.

One time a woman came to me in a wheelchair completely paralyzed with arthritis. After her first treatment she got out of the wheelchair and she is well and walking around today.

About six months ago I met her again and she was telling another woman in a wheelchair about the most wonderful pills she had taken for the same thing and how it had cured her. I just sat there and looked at her and then she said, "Of course, R. helped."

This seems to be the psychological pattern. When they are well they want to forget the whole thing. The doctor may save their life, and then they often try to cheat him out of the bill. It's human nature and not very nice at that.

248. I have been asked, "What is the difference between knowing and believing?" Knowing is an experience. Believing is something that could be. You may ask, I believe it but I don't accept it, but when you know, you absolutely believe. Your heart knows. Believing is of the mundane and knowing is of the supermundane.

I have worked with people who didn't believe in healing. They just wouldn't accept it; yet they were healed, and of very bad cases like cancer and leukemia and multiple sclerosis.

249. A bishop or minister who uses the Teaching in his church is doing a very good thing. As a matter of fact, in Trenton, New Jersey we had such a minister. Actually we were working with his congregation. His wife had multiple sclerosis so bad that she was crawling on her hands and knees. She couldn't stand up straight. In about two weeks she had a complete healing and both of their children had healings.

This man was on fire with the whole idea of healing and he preached from his pulpit about psychic energy and about the Mahatmas. He didn't go into details, but he would speak of the Hierarchy of Light. He worked on the basic theme that if we are Christians, we should be Christ-like and not gossipy or mean or dishonest to our brothers. He did very brilliant work for a time until some of his congregation began to go into a deeper study of the Teaching.

Suddenly he felt he was losing his church because some of his congregation were going into Theosophy and some into Agni Yoga. Some of the men who were very close to him were actually becoming disciples. Instead of letting them go on and progress, he tried to hold them back. Then, of course, his whole house of cards fell down around him, because no one can hold another person back. This is not right.

The man was told that if he would take healing into his church, they would turn away from three to five hundred people every Sunday. There would be no room for them. He refused. He wouldn't do it. Eventually, his church dwindled down to about fourteen people. The whole thing disintegrated. It was very tragic because this church was slated to do great things.

You see, in the ancient days of Greece, the church and healing were one. There was no exchange of money. It was all part of the religious scene. Then, in the days of the Romans, the church and healing became separated and the physicians took over and began to charge money and the whole thing changed. Now it's coming back into the church again and into religion where it should be.

250. There are many teachers. In fact, everyone you meet is your teacher, but there is only one Guru. When you work with the Guru, your whole body chemistry changes and you become more sensitive. For instance, a Stradivarius is a beautiful instrument and very sensitive and makes beautiful music. What you are doing is tuning yourself up to the concert pitch of a Stradivarius.

Medicine for a Yogi will not have the same effect as it does on other people. There are some people who for thirty years haven't even taken an aspirin, so any drug will give them a violent reaction. They can only be healed by psychic energy.

251. The chest that Roerich holds in his hands, in the portrait of Him done by his son Svetoslav, is symbolic of Pandora's Box. Once you have opened that box you have unleashed the elements within it and they can never be put back in. This symbology applies to Agni Yoga or any esoteric work. When you have gone to a certain point, you are holding a tiger by the tail and you can't let go or it will turn and devour you. Once you start down the occult road there is no stopping.

This is also true in healing. Once you start there is no stopping, because the more you give the more you receive. I once had a letter from Madame Roerich, in which she said I had gone beyond the point of no return in my healing work. She warned me never to stop healing or the energy would disintegrate me. You see, it's like water going through a pipe that's expanding, and once that pipe has expanded you dare not stop or you will be burned to a crisp.

The question has been asked, "When a person passes over, what happens to this great flow of psychic energy that has been utilized in healing?"

It goes with them, and then when they reincarnate that energy is added to them and they are brought back with more. Whatever you do here will go over with you and come back again with you and be added. There is never anything lost and there is no retrogression.

252. As Christ said, "They have eyes and they see not. They have ears and they hear not." Many years ago I went to hear Emmett Fox. He was a great healer and every Tuesday and Friday night he would give a healing in class.

One evening I was talking to this woman who had been going there for twelve years, and I said, "Mr. Fox is a very wonderful healer," and she said, "No, he isn't a healer." "But, my dear, he gives a healing every Tuesday and Friday night from the platform." She never heard it. For twelve years she sat there like a dunce and never heard it. They have ears and they hear not.

Emmett Fox would say to people, "Many of you have been coming here for years and years and years. This is the kindergarten of metaphysics. You should go on to high school and college, not stay in kindergarten the rest of your life." But they don't listen.

253. When they say in the Teaching, "We do not like cut flowers," it actually means that we shouldn't bring cut flowers in and leave them on the table to wither and die.

Flowers live only a short length of time to bring beauty to mankind, and by this sacrifice they become an individual soul on the wheel of transmigration.

Besides bringing beauty, all plants and leaves and flowers absorb poison and each flower has a healing quality. This is why we take flowers to the hospital.

The freesia is the most sacred and holy flower there is, and the rose is next. For instance, in the case of mental illness, if there is a freesia near the bed, no unwanted visitor can come in. It looks like a tiny little bell. They are pink and white and yellow.

The rose is very high in musk and the musk is the thing that saturates the air and will absorb any poisons in the room. This is why flowers die very quickly. They should be left in the room at night, but somebody told an old wives' tale that flowers take the oxygen out of the air, so the flowers are removed and the patient is getting the poison at night instead.

The lotus is pure and white and spotless, and it floats on the top of the water and the stem goes down deep into the mud and mire. The blossom remains untouched and this is a symbol of our consciousness, for as we live in the world of muck and mire, the spirit, like the lotus, is untouched.

Sacrifice

254. Sacrifice is one of the fastest ways to develop spiritually. When you can sacrifice your own pleasures, when you can sacrifice your time for other people, or sacrifice anything to help another individual, this is the fastest way. It is called selflessness. That and meditation will do it. If you never read another book or did another thing and you wanted to get closer and closer to this thing of wisdom and consciousness, that is the way do do it. It's very simple but very difficult.

255. One of the most touching stories of sacrifice I have ever heard was the story of Eddie Shebas, the senator in Cuba who fought Batista. This man was fighting for the poor people in Cuba. He gave something like four million dollars of his fortune. He sold his home, his art treasures, everything. He would speak on the air to these people and try to give them encouragement. He was absolutely fearless—a little bit of a guy with big thick glasses. He rode a bicycle and he would ride right up to a communist group and defy them.

One by one Batista would buy up the radio stations to shut him up, and this night he was broadcasting from the last station that was open to him. Just before his program ended he was handed a note which said this station was now owned by Batista and he could no longer speak to the people. So, at the end of the broadcast he said, "I have given my money. I have given my time, everything I have. I have only one thing left to give: my ideal and my life," and with that he shot himself. This was a sacrifice.

Joan of Arc did the same thing. She was promised absolute freedom if she would deny the voices that inspired her and she said, no, she would rather be burned at the stake than defile the voice of God. This was not suicide. This is an ideal and her death was a sacrifice.

And Socrates, too, said, "I will drink the hemlock rather than change my school to suit the people and thereby compromise my ideals."

This very act of Eddie Shebas brought about the defeat of Batista. You can kill a man but you can't kill his ideals. The idea was that he had nothing left to give but his life so he gave it and again I quote, "What greater love hath a man than to lay down his life for his brother?"

256. When the individuals who have been persecuted or killed come back, it's with an excellent karma because they have been sacrificed. For instance, the individuals who were burned in the ovens: true, this is tragic and sad and unjust, but they will come back to a better economic condition with more abilities, more advantages, more education, and have a much better place in life. It always works that way, because it's a sacrifice. Anyone who had been killed in war will be brought back into a better position than they were in in this life.

This takes away the whole fear of death. I think you people will agree with me that this great fear of death is a complete error because there is no death. It's a continuation of life. Yes, there is death to the physical body, but not to the consciousness, not to the soul or the spirit; that is eternal. Many of the Jewish churches and many of the Christian churches have held onto this misconception that you're going to rise from your rotten carcass and go to heaven. It's ridiculous. Many of the religions teach this to hold you through fear, the fear of "damnation forever" if you don't do what they tell you. But if God is as all-loving as they say He is, we should have no fear. There are two ways of working with people, either by love and faith and trust, or through fear and domination and control.

Boys killed in war do not have to wait in the Subtle World for their appointed time to die because this is a sacrifice, and so their return is speeded up. For instance, many of us remember past lives in which we have been killed and we came right back within a matter of two or three years or two or three months.

The church won't pick this up and give it out because then they couldn't control people through fear. This whole thing was given out centuries ago in the Upanishads and Vedas. The early Christian doctrine taught that the churches were for prayer and meditation and not for a man to get up and say, if you don't repent of your sins and do so and so, God will punish you.

One time I said to Swami Bodhinanda, "I hear so much about sin, what actually is it?" He said, "It's a sin that man is held in bondage by fear. This is not sin as we think of it, but it is regrettable that he is not a creature walking in light and illumination, because that is his right, his heritage and his privilege."

It was never meant that we should dominate another's spirit or consciousness. No two people can wear the same spiritual consciousness; they are all different, and any rabbi or priest or minister who gets up and says, "We are right and the rest are wrong," look out.

Run to the nearest exit because they don't know what they're talking about. The minute they say that, they cut themselves off from the complete source of God. All religions and creeds are right, but there is not one that is perfect. They all have their own way and they all reach the sunlit snows; however, they don't do it through fear and threatening, but by love, by understanding, by consciousness.

Beauty

257. In beauty there is God, and in beautiful things there is the refinement and cultivation of consciousness, and that is a cosmic law. All your creative people live in this world of beauty. The magic of creativity is in beauty and this moves the consciousness up to a higher level instead of being on a mundane level. Beauty is anything that will lift the consciousness out of the ego. When you hear beautiful music it takes you right out of yourself. When you see a beautiful painting you're taken right into it. It lifts you out of yourself, and your personality has soared into another sphere of existence. When you are reading poetry or prose and you come to a part that lifts the whole consciousness, you're experiencing beauty that is literally magic.

Mr. F. in Taos said to me, "I have met several of your disciples and all of them have a light that emanates from their skin." This is true of all the disciples, and that light is the light from within, and this is the beauty that is brought through the consciousness. Children feel it and animals feel it, and they are attracted to it.

This is the thing that bridges the gap in age because the consciousnesses meet. No matter how old or how young people are, if that consciousness of beauty is there, there is no gap. Beauty is limitless. It's a form of magic. Something magical takes place and suddenly your spirit soars into infinity. This is the thing that gets you off the ground. For instance, if you're writing you're not sitting there banging the typewriter, you're some place else. Inspiration is flowing through you and this great beauty is responding, and truth is also part of that beauty. This is why you are constantly told, "discrimination, discrimination," because in discrimination there is great beauty.

258. Ugliness of thought and surroundings prevent you from living in the Subtle World. Master R. always said, "The more beautiful your surroundings are, the finer your quality will be because

you will become attuned to that beauty. You can live in absolute beauty and luxury as long as you're not attached to it and it doesn't own you. The most important thing in the world, next to God Consciousness, is to live in beauty." Things don't necessarily need to be expensive, but they should be of good quality and have nice line and color and be in good taste.

I always encourage people to start collecting art because this is a source of great beauty. One very fine art collection belonged to a man who worked in an office for sixty-five dollars a week. Every year he went abroad and traveled by bicycle and everywhere he went he bought paintings and sculpture. After ten years his collection was worth a hundred and sixty-five thousand dollars. He had very good taste, and he would buy what he could afford and then later trade it for something better.

One of the great Russian collections belonged to a young prince who had no money, a friend of Master R.'s. He started buying the work of the early Russian painters, and when the Communists took over he had one of the finest art collections in Russia which he had built out of virtually nothing. It doesn't take fortunes. It takes intelligence and diligence and the desire to do it.

Every painting that you look at in a museum is absorbed into your consciousness and it will remain in your memory for all the rest of your lives. The word "museum" is from the Greek, meaning the "house of muses." Whenever you go to a museum, think that you are going to the house of the gods and godesses. If you think of painting and poetry and music in this way, it will penetrate into your consciousness at a new level and become a tremendously beautiful experience. As Buddha said, "All around you is this light and beauty and happiness that are beyond the wildest dreams of man, and all you need do is reach out and touch it and it is yours."

259. A spiritual experience is anything that will lift you out of yourself. For instance, a young boy was working for us, and I sent him up to the shrine room for something and he fainted. I went up and revived him and I said, "Has anything like this ever happened to you before?" and he said, "Yes, once I went into the Episcopal Church at Christmas, and the flowers and the altar were so beautiful and I fainted." The beauty lifted him and his consciousness went right out so that he actually had a spiritual experience at that moment.

260. There is a beautiful church in Los Angeles on the corner of Normandy and Pico. It is Byzantine Greek, and so beautiful and so perfect and so exquisite that when you walk into it you'll say, "Oh, my God." When you enter, your spirit feels suddenly lifted.

As I've told you many times, Roerich always taught, "Through beauty you can lift the consciousness.'' You can do more through beauty than any other way. We can read books, we can hear the word for hours, but beauty speaks to the hearts of men and lifts the whole consciousness. Music, too, will do what nothing else can.

Another interesting thing about this church was that the man who dreamed of building it was Greek Orthodox, and he died before it was ready to be built. But his wife, who was a Mormon, saw that the church was built and paid for because this was what he wanted. She could easily have said, no, I want this for my church.

261. There is a story of a Dutch family in Africa. They were rather old to be parents, but the mother wanted a beautiful child. Neither one of them were very beautiful people, but she kept praying and looking at pictures of beautiful children, and when the child was born it didn't look like either of them. It was a raving beauty. Evidently she drew that spirit to her. Now, people who are attractive have earned that through their consciousness, and the more beautiful they are the more wonderful the consciousness has been, but what they do with it in this life is another story.

They can wreck it with their ego. There is a movie star who is a great, great beauty but she's destroyed the whole thing through her desires and senses.

Many people rely on their beauty. There was a man whom we did business with and he had a terrible nose. It was huge and quite ugly, but he was the most charming, considerate person you'd ever want to meet. Everybody loved him, and then he had his nose fixed and he was very handsome. And do you know, he lost all his personality and became a big bore. This often happens.

Service

262. You can return any time you want to the planet you came from, but many people—when they pass over and see where they can work best—will offer to come back. Service is the whole key to everything.

There is the story of this man who was lying in the daisy field looking at the clouds when all of a sudden one of the clouds descended to the daisy field and a little dwarf was standing on the cloud. He bid the man come over to the cloud and get on, and then he showed him how to balance himself with his solar plexus, and the cloud took off and went to a great building in which there were many men, women and children of all races, colors, creeds and religions. There were great halls and tables, and the dwarf took him inside where he was given a beautiful white book with gold lettering around the edges, whereupon they went back to the cloud, descended, and the man went back to his daisy field. The cloud disappeared and he opened the book, but there was only one page in the book and on that page but one word, and that word was SERVICE. This is actually the whole reason for our being here; service to one another.

But, if you are of service and all the time are thinking, "I am doing this to be of service," you are defeating yourself. You do it because it is there to be done without thought of how it will benefit you to have done this. It is a very fine line.

263. Any service you perform, even if you are paid for it, is a service, but if you hate what you are doing and are only doing it to collect a pay check, you are not serving.

People often ask me, "How can I serve?" Teaching is a wonderful way of serving and so is medicine. Doctors, nurses and healers are some of the greatest servants of humanity. The Teachings say, "To take away pain from another person is the fastest way to God Consciousness." The book, *Psychic Healing*, (*The Science of Psychic Healing*, by Ramacharaka) is a wonderful book and explains all the facets of healing. Then all you have to do is set up your shop by the side of the road and the Hierarchy will send you the people. Some people are more skilled in healing than others, but as you develop spiritually, your healing skills will develop, too. You are nothing but an instrument, and the healing power is through God or the Law of Nature. You merely offer yourself as a channel and direct this energy to the individual. It's the Hierarchy working through you, so you are not doing it.

If you have a neighbor who is ill, go and offer help. Ask if you can bring in some food or whatever is needed. Or, if someone is in difficulty, ask if you can help. Sometimes it's enough to just listen to them.

There are many ways to be of service, and when you offer yourself in service to the Hierarchy, They use you, but never unless you offer. All disciples offer immediately, and often students do too.

Many people come into the Teaching for various reasons. Sometimes they think they will use the Teaching, but I have to chuckle because the Teaching always turns around and uses them. You see, it's much bigger than we are and once you open that power, They use you.

264. The Hierarchy will never ask you to do anything you are not capable of doing. If They say this is an assignment and you are ready to do it, you are ready. Many times people will say, "I don't feel I am prepared." I know; I was guilty of saying that very thing. But They said, "If We did not think you were ready, We wouldn't ask you." So you shouldn't have this false modesty. If you are asked to do it, They know, and you do it.

Many times during the day you may be there in body but your spirit is withdrawn. When you offer yourself in service to the Hierarchy, They use you; They use your energy even though you may not be aware of it. For instance, in healing sometimes I am not aware of the particular place where I am doing the healing, but the individual who is sick will often see me and then recognize me later on when we meet.

265. The term "common labor" means service to humanity in any way, shape, or form. All the wisdom and knowledge in the world is useless unless you can put it to work. The whole idea is that if we can make this a better world for just one person we have not lived in vain. Otherwise, we are cluttering up the Earth with our bodies and just taking up space. If we can extend this idea many times over then we are really accomplishing something.

An example of this is found in one of the most magnificent gestures ever made. Nikola Tesla developed alternating current and sold it to Westinghouse for a million dollars plus a royalty on each kilowatt hour used. Later on Mr. Westinghouse came to him and said, "Mr. Tesla, we have signed the contract, and we owe you the money. You can collect it, but it will ruin the company. We cannot continue AC current under these terms." Tesla said, "Give me the contract." He tore it up and threw it into the wastebasket. He said it was more important that people have AC current than that he have thirty-two million dollars. He really justified his existence, and when he died he left over a thousand inventions to the world.

Likewise, Roerich left eight thousand paintings when he died. He wrote twenty-eight books, was an archeologist, an anthropologist, and founded cultural organizations all over the world. He created the wonderful Pact and Banner of Peace, and he was a Teacher. He accepted this great responsibility and accomplished the impossible.

266. In Rome there is a group of businessmen who at certain times of the year, like Christmas or Thanksgiving, put on monks' robes with a cowl that covers their faces, and they go out among the poor and give money.

In New York City I once knew an Oxford Don who was a very fine Theosophist and his dedication to service was to leave a bushel basket of groceries at the door of the poor people, ring the bell, and run like hell. But, as he got older he could no longer negotiate the stairs or run fast enough, so he solicited four or five people to help him. I helped him do these things for about a year and a half and nobody knew about it, not even his wife. After he died, I talked with her and she said she never knew.

If you are doing a special work to help people, do it in secret. This is like interest in the bank. If you go to the bank and draw out a dollar every day, you end up with no interest. If you go around and boast about all the good things you have done and let your ego run rampant, you lose the interest and your good deeds are worthless, completely worthless; but if you do it in secret the good is multiplied tenfold. Remember Shakespeare's words in *The Merchant of Venice*, "It is blest, it is twice blest for those who give and those who receive." This is a cosmic law; this is karma.

267. We are in bondage in our physical bodies. We have aches and pains, desires, lust, anger, hatred, jealousy; in fact, everything from the world of desire. Even the desire to become a Mahatma will defeat your purpose. As Buddha said, "When you become desireless, then all things are open to you." As you develop you will "Become" by your thinking. This doesn't mean you should sit and twiddle your thumbs, but you must get out and work. Your duty is to serve humanity.

At one of the Ashrams in India, the Guru would send two of his students to the kitchen to do the cooking while he was conducting classes for the others. These men thought they were missing something and not developing, and so they went to the Guru and protested. He told them, "Since you are giving up something for your brothers, this pushes you way ahead. Instead of sitting in the classroom and getting something for yourselves, you are serving others, therefore you will evolve faster than the men sitting in the class just listening. As you serve, so you develop spiritually."

268. When you offer yourself for service you will not necessarily know what you are being used for, but it's not as important that we know how we are being used by the Hierarchy as it is that we offer ourselves to be used.

For instance, there was a man in Canada who was telling me this story. He said he had borrowed a very expensive car to use to go and see his girl. He was intending to give her an engagement ring and ask her to marry him, but as he was driving to her house the car caught on fire. He threw up the hood and was trying to smother the fire with his coat, and then he was putting it out with his hands and they were horribly burned. He was feeling very badly because he felt responsible for the car.

This happened in a small village up near Ottawa with only about three or four hundred people, and this man, beautifully dressed all in grey, suddenly appeared and took both his hands in his and said, "You will be all right, just relax." He looked at his hands and there was no burn and no blisters, and then the man disappeared. No one knew him or could find him. This sort of thing happens very often.

In Italy they were telling me this story that happened during World War II when the Germans were there. They were having a terrible time in the battlefield and there were no doctors. The wounded were coming in by the truckload and the doctors were all up at the front. This woman was working alone and so she went into the chapel and prayed, and when she came out there stood this elegantly dressed gentleman who said he was a doctor from Rome. So she put him to work, and he worked there for three days until the other doctors came back from the front lines, and then he disappeared. And when they tried to find out who he was they found that no doctor had been sent from Rome. She said while he was there it was miraculous what he did with the patients and the people that were healed. This would be a Mahatma.

You see, the minute you are a disciple one of your subtle bodies is in Shambhala. There are seven bodies and your physical body is only one of them. One subtle body can be divided into seven subtle bodies. This is why an individual can be seen in several different places at the same time. In the case of HPB, one of her bodies was kept in Shambhala to facilitate the link the Hierarchy had with her. They used that body as a contact.

In the same way, at night when you go to sleep, your subtle body divides into several different bodies and they are sent to different places. You may go to three, four, five, six or seven places at the same time.

Devotion

269. Can an abundance of one quality make up for the lack of another quality?

Yes, if you have an abundance of devotion, it doesn't matter if you are a stumblebum and stupid and everything else, you will still get it (enlightenment), but if you're brilliant and have no devotion, you will get nowhere. That is the trick—this thing of devotion. It is the armor of the individual. If you have no devotion you can't get anywhere, period. I don't mean devotion to me, but devotion to the Teaching and to Roerich. Devotion means listening to what I tell you when you ask for advice.

270. Remember how few disciples Christ had? When He was in the garden of Gethsemane and the soldiers came and asked which is the Christ, they all denied any knowledge of Him. This was their weakness.

The same thing happened with Apollonius of Tyana. When he came to the Roman gates he had thirty-four staunch disciples. A soldier came out and said, "The Emperor is going to arrest you," and suddenly thirty-three disciples had pressing business at home.

He was taken in and put in chains. The Emperor wanted to destroy him, but Apollonius was so brilliant and so skillful in his replies that the people demanded he be allowed to go free.

When people are put in a bad position where they must choose between staying or taking flight, they will nearly always take flight.

271. There is this story about a poor woman who worked in a cabbage patch and all her life she had been praying for a Buddha. This prayer was ever on her lips, "Bring me a Buddha. I wish I had a Buddha for my shrine." Then one day, as she was working among her cabbages, she came upon this beautiful golden Buddha with amethyst eyes and a beautiful jewell on the forehead. She was delighted and ran to put it on her shrine. Every day, morning, noon and night, she would go to the shrine to do her prayers. But as the winter came, and then the spring, and she had to till her ground and plant her seeds and take care of them, she neglected her shrine and didn't go near it. The next year at about the same time she was in her cabbage patch at the same spot where she had found her Buddha. Suddenly she remembered and rushed down to her shrine, but the Buddha was gone because of neglect. You may have a treasure, but if you neglect your treasure you will lose it.

Neglect in your spiritual life does not come when things are going badly for you and you are working against tremendous odds, but when all goes well and you are very successful, then you must hang on with everything you've got or you'll lose it.

272. Any individual who is sincere and devoted, no matter what their religion or philosophy is and if they have an absolute purity of knowing the truth about themselves, will have a good life. But very few have this ability because it takes terrific discrimination.

People may go to church and be good people, they pay their debts, they don't gossip, they do their duty. But this isn't enough. Everyone should do that. You need to do more. You need to dedicate yourself to do the work of the Lord out in the world.

There is a story about this playwright who had a child with water on the brain. His doctor told him that if it didn't gel in three or four days it never would and the baby would be an idiot.

It was the fourth day and the father went to a specialist and said, "I must have the best medical attention, no matter what the cost."

The specialist said, "I know the case and from a medical point of view it's hopeless, but I'll tell you one doctor who may help you."

"I'll fly him here. I'll do anything."

The specialist said, "This won't even cost you a nickle. If you dedicate yourself to the Lord's work and pray to the Lord and offer yourself sincerely to do His work, I'm sure the child will be healed."

So the father prayed all night long and the next morning the child was healed with no brain damage.

Then he wrote a great play and it was performed at the Roerich Master Institute. I went to see it and found he had deleted the whole thing of the child. The play was a flop because he brought the story of this man and woman and child up to the point of the healing and stopped. He was afraid somebody would laugh at him.

He went to Hollywood to work in pictures and every place he went it was failure, failure, until he finally gave up.

Once we have touched the hem of the robe and dedicated ourself, we have to follow through. If we say, "I dedicate myself next time around," it doesn't work. This is why Roerich always said, "Never take a vow." The best thing to say is, "I will try and do this," but never take a vow. Do the things you are capable of. Don't lose faith with yourself. When we make this world a better place for one person we have not lived in vain.

Striving and Solemnity

273. Striving in the Teaching means that you are trying. It means you want more information and experience. You want to throw yourself deeply into it. You want to be dedicated, to give your life for it.

You can't strive with ego. It's impossible. The "I" should want to know what it can give not what it can receive. I was in Mexico one time and during a meditation I got this beautiful phrase which I want to pass on to you, "We do not teach, but we share our knowledge."

274. If we are satisfied with what we see and hear, we are wearing blinders. We must have divine discontent. The more divine discontent you have the harder you will strive, and the more knowledge and wisdom you will achieve.

Divine discontent is the best thing in the world. When we are content and smug about ourselves, that's the end of our spiritual growth and development. You should constantly say, "I want wisdom. I want knowledge. These are the most important things, and I will never be satisfied with what I have." We should want these things as badly as the man on the desert who is dying of thirst wants water.

275. Striving is good because it will make you go forward. Striving is like having a dream. If you have a dream, you will go on to accomplish it. If you have no dream, you have no direction. Many people have lost their dream, and for them I feel very sad. Always remember, the impossible dream is the most important thing. No matter how impossible it is, you will realize it, but it takes courage and you have to fight for it.

Like great artists who will starve to death in order to paint. I was talking to an artist in New York recently who said, "New York is beating me. Shall I go home or shall I stay?" I said, "Do you want to be an artist?" He said, "Yes." I said, "Well then, stay and starve if necessary, but paint. Go home, and you've lost your dream and you'll end up being a nothing."

People will tell you there's no room at the top. Believe me, there's all kinds of room at the top, but you have to fight like hell to get there if that's what you want. If that's not what you want then don't bother, but that's your rightful place in the sun.

To illustrate this, there was a little girl in Ohio who dreamed that one day she would marry a Maharaja in India and live in great splendor. She had no more chance of going to India than that table, but suddenly a series of events changed her life and she found herself in India married to a great Maharaja and she is now a Maharani. She believed the impossible, and the moment you believe, it is possible.

You must never think that you can't. In the New Age School in Texas we have the word "CAN'T" and the "T" is on a trap door and the kids knock the "T" down and then it spells CAN. I would like to remove the words "can't" and "impossible" from the dictionary because they're stumbling blocks.

276. When you do something wrong just say, "I've done

something wrong, I'm not going to do it again," and drop it. "It's an experience and I'm going to learn from this and not dwell on it, but leave it; therefore, I ask God to forgive me and I ask the person I have injured to forgive me and that's it."

There was a man in Cuba, a leading politician, and like many politicians, he lied and slandered and misrepresented and ruined many people. Later on his conscience got the better of him and, being a Catholic, he went to his priest and said, "Father, I have hurt many people and lied and injured them and it's bothering me. What shall I do?"

The priest said, "Take a feather pillow, go up on the highest mountain, cut the pillow open and let all the feathers fly in the wind, and when you have done this come back and see me."

The man thought, "This is easy." He went away and did as he was told and when he returned, the priest said, "Now, go out and pick up every feather." "But that's impossible," the man said, "I can't do it. The wind has carried them here and there and all over." And the Father said, "What you have done is also impossible to correct, but what you can do is go to the few remaining people you have injured and beg their forgiveness."

When you do something wrong, go to the individual and ask for forgiveness. If they forgive you, you are released from that karma. You still have to pay the karma of the action, but not for the wrong you have done to the individual. No matter what you have done, no matter how terrible it is, if you sincerely ask for forgiveness in your heart, you are forgiven, not by a priest or rabbi or minister but in your heart by that cosmic law. No one can do it for you for a fee; only you can do it for yourself.

If you can ask someone to forgive you this makes you a stronger person, a better person in their eyes, and they will never forget it. It takes a big person to say, "I'm sorry, I was wrong, forgive me." Nothing can upset you and keep you from doing this but your ego, and that is the whole essence of metaphysics. It takes selflessness and meditation and commitment and self examination and more meditation.

277. It's not that the use of alcohol or tobacco or meat is a sin, but as you meditate and strive, your body chemistry changes and you cannot tolerate these things any more. If you are a meat eater, don't suddenly give it up or you will become ill, but if you no longer like it, it has given you up and this is fine. You must always remember: it is not as important what you put into the mouth as what comes out.

278. You know you are fulfilling the higher will by being unselfish, by thinking of others and not yourself. The idea of

selflessness is to think of the other person to such an extent that you don't count for anything. You mean absolutely nothing. You have no desire and your ego doesn't want to be fed. You think only of the needs of others.

But, if you're going to do a good deed and then say, oh boy, am I getting good karma for that, it won't work. This is no good.

279. The Mahatmas have individual personalities just as you and I have as a result of all our past lives. They have solemnity, but they also have a terrific sense of humor which they never lose. The idea is to not become a fanatic. In many of the good monasteries, if one of the monks becomes too serious or gets a little pompous or a little precious, the Swami will send him out into the world until he gets his sense of humor back.

What is meant by solemnity is: when you are working with the Teaching, you are completely serious and at one with it, and give it your undivided attention and reverence. It doesn't mean you should be light-minded about it. Actually, Yoga is opening Pandora's Box. As I've told you many times, it's like holding a tiger by the tail, and you can't let go or it will turn and devour you. There is no stopping once you start, so this is why They say be sure you know what you are doing or leave it alone. There is no danger in yoga whatsoever, unless your ego becomes so involved and inflated that you can't handle it. The other danger is breathing exercises. Many people go off on their own, read a book and apply it to themselves. You can't do that because there are no two people alike.

The same is true with disciples. We will tell one disciple one thing, and that is only for them because of their development. Another disciple we will tell something completely different, because that's their development and no two are completely alike. Now, when they get together one disciple will say, "My Guru said this," and the other disciple will say, "But he didn't tell me that," and away they go until soon they have lost the whole quality and essence of what they were told. This is why if you are told something, guard it well; it's for you and you alone.

This is true of any creative thought or idea, the moment you talk about it, the idea becomes dissipated. The more you talk about it the more dissipated it becomes; it gets weaker and weaker, until you never do it. But if you hold this idea or thought as a secret or tell someone who is sympathetic to your work and who will then pray and work with you, you can do it. If you have one person who believes in you, you can do the impossible.

If you have a bad dream about someone, tell it because this breaks it immediately. If you have a good dream about an individual—something very good and wonderful—don't tell it, because you want it to happen, and it may come about.

There was a playwright in London who wrote a play called *The Cobra*. At the time he was doing this the very same play was being produced in America. They both opened on the same night with the same story almost exactly word for word. There was a big lawsuit charging plagiarism and then they found that the playwrights had never met. They traced it to both men having been guests at the same party in Paris where they heard this story about a cobra in India. They both went their separate ways and wrote the very same play.

280. When we are striving in any particular direction it's a very serious business. To have a good sense of humor is wonderful and very helpful, but the solemnity is in your prayer, in your mediation, in your study and in your striving. The rest of the time, use your sense of humor. The ancient Chinese medicine teaches that laughter will cure any disease, because your blood flows, you're completely relaxed, and you're enjoying everything.

In solemnity, too, there is joy. When you are working and striving with this thing of God, there is great joy, because you are part of it. But it cannot be done in halfwayness. Many people go into something halfway because somebody else did it or because it's the smart thing to do. This is not solemnity and you are not going to get anything out of it. It's what you put into it and not what you get out of it that counts. If you take your solemnity and devotion and striving and love with you into any church or temple or synagogue or philosophy, you will go away with much more than if you take nothing. If you take nothing with you, you go away empty-handed.

We all kid around and have a lot of fun, but when we are working in the class or with people individually, then it is a very serious thing and all kidding is set aside. This is all part of this thing of solemnity. You may be very, very pure and have a very pure motive, but if you have no sense of humor, then you are out of balance. That is why we say joy, joy, joy. Everything is joy. It doesn't mean you're going ha, ha, ha, but it means you have joy in your heart. You have joy for God, you have joy for music, you have joy for literature, you have joy for your loved ones, you have joy for all of nature, the wind and the rain. It doesn't mean you should go around with a long face, but you should enjoy everything that God has put before you: beauty, birds, the wind, the beautiful trees, the mountains, and when you look at all these things there should be great joy in your heart.

Subject Index